Ken

The Menopause

Karen Lloyd.

The Menopause

Mary Anderson MB, ChB, FRCOG

faber and faber
LONDON·BOSTON

First published in 1983
by Faber and Faber Limited
3 Queen Square London WC1N 3AU
Reprinted 1983, 1984
Printed in Great Britain by
Redwood Burn Ltd., Trowbridge, Wiltshire
All rights reserved

British Library Cataloguing in Publication Data

Anderson, Mary
The menopause.
1. Menopause
I. Title
612'.665   RG186

ISBN 0–571–13071–2

...The best is yet to be,
The last of life, for which the first was made...

ROBERT BROWNING, 'Rabbi Ben Ezra'

Contents

List of illustrations and tables   *page* 8
Author's preface   9
Acknowledgements   11
1 Anatomy: the structure of the female organs   13
2 Physiology: how the female organs function   22
3 The menopause: what it is and why it happens   31
4 Menopausal symptoms and signs   37
5 Treatment of the menopause   59
6 Questions which arise at the menopause   81
7 Personal viewpoint   95
8 The male 'menopause'   98
   Glossary   103
   Suggested further reading   109
   Index   110

Illustrations

1	External genitalia	*page* 15
2	Internal genitalia	17
3	Ovaries and Fallopian tubes	19
4	Breast structure	21
5	Control of menstruation	23

Tables

1	Summary of events leading to menstruation	26
2	Symptoms of prolapse	42
3	Oestrogens in common usage	62
4	Combined oestrogen-progestogen preparations	66
5	Continuous hormone replacement therapy	67
6	Oestrogen-testosterone preparations	70

Author's preface

When it was suggested to me that I should write a small book on the menopause for the non-medical reader, I was hesitant. Surely there was enough available literature on the subject? A search through these books and pamphlets showed, however, that they tended to be written either in a somewhat racy anecdotal style – not everyone's choice – or in an oversimplified, somewhat condescending way, which must have proved irritating, or at least inadequate, for many readers.

This book is an attempt to explain the facts of the menopause, its whys and wherefores, the bodily changes which take place and the symptoms which may (or, more importantly, may not) occur. It attempts to suggest what can be done by women to accept and to cope with this landmark in their lives, helped by drugs where appropriate but always by guidance and understanding.

My qualifications for writing such a book are that as a woman and a gynaecologist I am frequently asked by my patients to explain 'the menopause' to them. I am impressed by their response to a matter-of-fact and not oversimplified explanation based on medical knowledge and scientific facts rather than a breezy journalistic approach.

Whether I will be successful in the written word is for the interested reader to judge.

Acknowledgements

This book was written at the suggestion of Miss P. Downie, Medical and Nursing Editor, Faber and Faber, and my thanks are due to her for much encouragement, assistance and constructive criticism.

The book is dedicated to friend and colleague alike since much of what is written results from mutual discussion and understanding, which I freely acknowledge.

M.A., 1983

1 · Anatomy: the structure of the female organs

Every medical student knows that he must learn about the structure of the body and its components and the way they function before he can progress to a study of illness or variations from normal with any hope of understanding. The same guiding principle must be used in a book such as this. Every medical student equally knows how boring the study of anatomy and physiology can be (but need not be), but for the purposes of this book boredom can be avoided by presenting the facts briefly and basically with illustrations to help.

The female genital organs consist of the external genitalia which are the structures of the *vulva*, and the internal genitalia which are the *vagina*, the *uterus*, the *tubes* and the *ovaries*.

The vulva (Fig. 1)

This comprises several structures which surround the entrance to the vagina.

1. *The labia majora* ('large lips'): These are two large folds of skin filled with fat and containing hair follicles and sweat glands. They vary in size, becoming smaller after the menopause. In front they merge into the pad of fat which lies over the pubic bone. This is known as the *mons pubis* or *veneris* (in ancient anatomical terms it was called the Mount of Venus) and is covered by skin and hairs. Behind, the labia majora become thinner and merge into the 'wedge' of

muscular tissue which lies between the back border of the vagina and the opening of the bowel (the *anus*).

2. *The labia minora* ('small lips'): These are two smaller folds of pink skin lying immediately on either side of the entrance to the vagina (known as the *vestibule*), enclosed by the labia majora. They contain very little fat and no hair, but many blood vessels. They are separated by a narrow groove from the inner surfaces of the labia majora—which, unlike their outer surfaces, do not contain hair.

3. *The clitoris* is the female equivalent of the male penis. It is about 2.5cm long (this is variable) and consists of erectile tissue which becomes engorged with blood during sexual excitement and can lead to orgasm when directly stimulated. It is surrounded by the front part of the labia majora which split into two folds to encircle it (Fig. 1).

Just below the clitoris is the *urethral* opening through which urine is passed from the bladder.

4. *The hymen* is the thin, incomplete membrane which surrounds the opening to the vagina (which is sometimes referred to as the *introitus*).

Only tags of this membrane remain after sexual intercourse has begun or even following the use of tampons. These tags are known as *carunculae myrtiformes*.

Round either side of the introitus and outside the hymen are two collections of erectile tissue which, like the clitoris, fill with blood during sexual excitement. They are called the *vestibular bulbs*. At their lower end on either side are two small pea-sized glands with ducts opening on the surface just outside the lower end of the hymen and inside the lower end of the labia minora. They secrete mucus to provide lubrication, particularly during inter-

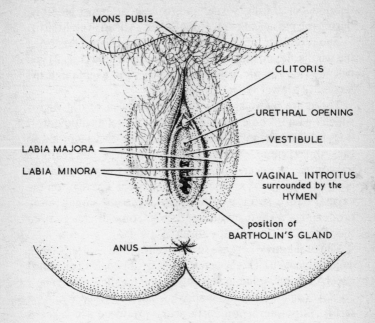

Fig. 1   External genitalia

course, and are called *Bartholin's glands* after the 17th-century Danish anatomist who first described them.

The internal genitalia (Fig. 2)

The remainder of the female pelvic organs are inside the body and consist of the following:

THE VAGINA

This is basically a hollow muscular tube about 9cm long leading from the vestibule below to the uterus above. Normally the front and back walls lie together in apposition but the vagina is lined by skin containing many folds and so it is capable of considerable stretching as occurs when inserting tampons or during sexual intercourse or, most notably, during the passage downwards of a baby's head in childbirth.

The *cervix* (or 'neck of the womb') projects into the top of the vagina. If you look at the pelvis from the side (Fig. 2) you will see that the *bladder* lies in front of the vagina and the *rectum* (or lower bowel) is behind it.

There are many blood vessels in the wall of the vagina which again become distended during sexual excitement. It does not contain any glands to produce its own secretion so that the common term 'vaginal discharge' is really a misnomer. It does, however, collect secretions from the glands of the cervix and also from the 'wear and tear' on the vaginal skin's surface cells which gradually slough away producing a certain amount of debris. Some discharge from the vagina is, therefore, entirely normal.

The breakdown of these surface cells produces a substance called glycogen. This is acted upon by a bacillus (or germ) which normally inhabits the vagina and is called *Döderlein's bacillus* (again after the man who first described it). As a result of this interaction, lactic acid is produced which keeps the environment of the vagina acid and prevents infection from any outside contamination.

After the menopause the lining skin of the vagina becomes thin (see p. 39) and this process of lactic-acid production does not readily occur. As a result, inflammation of the vagina ('vaginitis') may result with actual infection.

THE UTERUS AND CERVIX

The *uterus* (or womb) is a hollow, pear-shaped organ lying above the vagina within the pelvis proper. It measures approximately 7.6cm in length, 5cm in width at its widest part and weighs about 60g. It has thick muscular walls about 1.5cm in depth and its cavity is normally just a slit but capable of enormous distension such as is demanded of it during pregnancy.

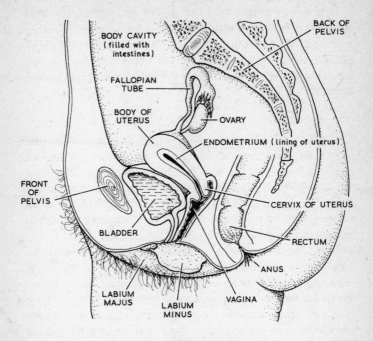

Fig. 2   Internal genitalia

The main bulk of the uterus above the vagina is termed the *body* of the uterus, and the narrower portion projecting into the vagina, the neck or *cervix*. This is the part of the uterus that is so accessible to examination and from which smear tests are taken to study its covering cells and look for signs of actual or potential abnormalities, mainly cancer.

The cavity of the uterus is lined by special tissue, known as endometrium, which thickens during a monthly cycle and is then shed off during menstruation if a pregnancy has not occurred. The basis of these important changes is described in Chapter 2.

It is worth noting that the uterus and cervix are held supported in their position by fan-shaped tissue on either side which spreads out to the muscles on the side walls of the pelvis. Weakening of these supports in older women may lead to a slipping downwards of the uterus and cervix known as *prolapse*.

THE TUBES AND OVARIES (Fig. 3)

The tubes, or *Fallopian tubes* to give them their full title (after the anatomist who first described them – Fallopius –in the 16th century), are two hollow tubes about 10cm long which project out from either side of the upper part of the body of the uterus. At their outer ends they hang over the ovaries with finger-like processes and therefore provide a connecting link between the ovaries and the cavity of the uterus. These finger-like processes, or *fimbriae* as they are called, pick up the egg produced on the surface of the ovary. The egg is then carried along the tube helped by the tube's muscular activity and by the special cells lining it, which have hair-like projections on their surface to waft the egg along. Fertilisation of the egg takes place within the tube and the fertilised egg is then carried to the cavity of the uterus where it implants in the specialised lining now known as *decidua*.

The *ovaries* are two almond-shaped bodies, whitish in colour with a corrugated appearance. In middle life they are approximately 3cm long, 2cm broad and weigh about 6g. After the menopause the ovaries diminish in size and may become very tiny, wrinkled organs in old age. The outer coat of each ovary is called the *cortex* and is the functioning portion of the organ, containing the egg cells embedded in a layer of cells called the *stroma*. The outer covering is a tight coat called the *tunica albuginea*.

In the centre of each ovary is the portion known as the *medulla* which carries the blood vessels and nerves of the glands.

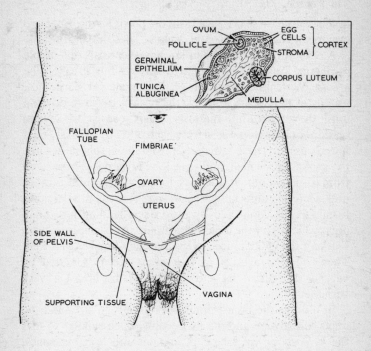

Fig. 3   Ovaries and Fallopian tubes. The inset shows the structure of an ovary

The ovaries are really the equivalent of the testicles in the male. Not only do they produce eggs during the reproductive years – they contain about 200 000 egg cells at the onset of maturity – but they also secrete the female sex hormones. This process is described on page 24.

The breasts (Fig. 4)

Some considerable distance from the pelvis lie the other two organs which are typical of the female. These are the breasts.

As everyone knows, the infant breast consists of a nipple projecting from the pinkish area surrounding it called the *areola*. With the production of the female sex hormones, usually at the age of 10 to 12, the breasts begin to develop until they reach full maturity. They consist of several sections or lobes separated from each other by a thin sheet of fibrous tissue. These radiate out from the areola rather like the spokes of a wheel, and each lobe is therefore separated from its neighbour. Inside each lobe are little collections of milk-secreting units known as *alveoli*. These consist of milk-forming cells connected by little ducts leading into main ducts which carry the milk to the nipple. As can be seen from Figure 4 the appearance is very like the branches of a tree. These basic structures of the breast are surrounded by varying degrees of fat and the size of the breast is very variable.

In old age the breast diminishes greatly in size, and the ducts, the alveoli and the fat become much smaller so that the breasts are no longer prominent and firm but small, rather wrinkled and drooping.

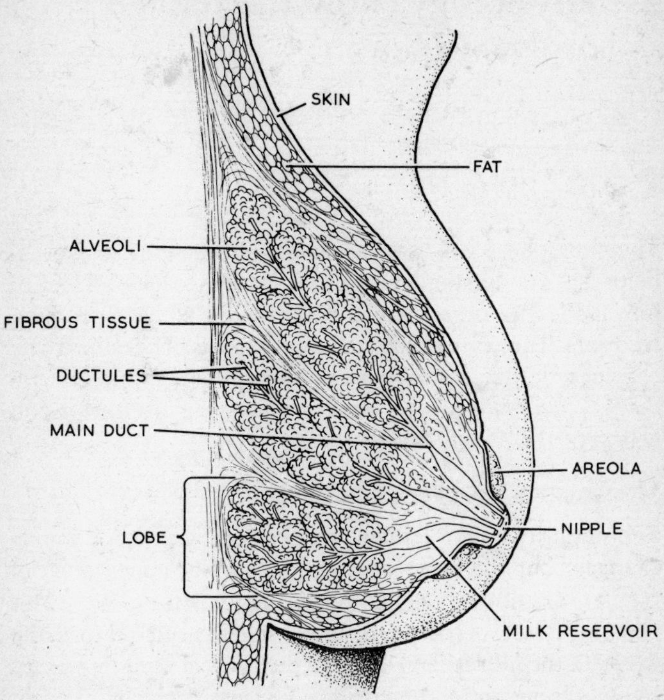

Fig. 4   The structure of a breast

2 · Physiology: how the female organs function

The menopause is a time of change of function, so again it helps one's understanding of these changes to have an idea of how the female organs function during the active reproductive years. There are really two main aspects of function to be considered: first, *menstruation*, which is closely linked with *the function of the ovaries*, and secondly, the production and action of the *female hormones*.

Menstruation and ovarian function

Full maturity of the female is associated with many bodily changes, but the most obvious one is the appearance of regular monthly vaginal bleeding – *menstruation*. This bleeding is not, of course, from the vagina itself but from the cavity of the uterus, and denotes the cyclical shedding of the cavity's lining, the endometrium. The age at which this event begins is variable but in the Western world is between 12 and 15 years, at the time of puberty; and the onset of menstruation is known as the *menarche*. At the other end of life, again at a variable age but approximately between 45 and 55 years, menstruation stops and this event is called the *menopause* (from the Greek – *men*: month; *pausis*: cessation).

The control of menstruation and the cyclical events which also occur in the ovary are shown in a simplified diagram (Fig. 5). Summarised, the complex train of events is as follows:

1. A portion of the brain called the *hypothalamus*

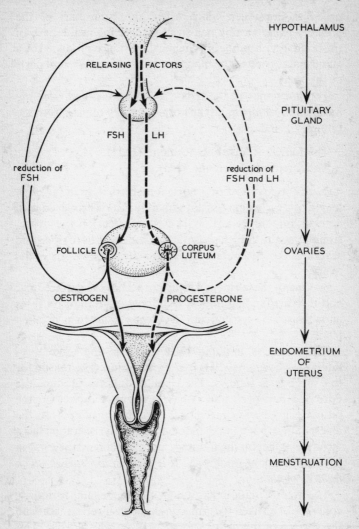

Fig. 5 Control of menstruation

produces hormones which affect the front part of the *pituitary gland* – a tiny pea-sized gland lying in the base of the brain. (A *hormone* is a chemical substance produced by a gland and carried in the bloodstream to affect different parts of the body.)

The hormones of the hypothalamus are called *releasing factors or hormones* and the hormones they release from the pituitary gland are:

The follicle-stimulating hormone (FSH)
The luteinising hormone (LH)

2. In the first part of a normal menstrual cycle (average length of a cycle being 28 days) mainly FSH is produced with a small amount of LH. FSH has an effect on the ovary, stimulating the 'follicles' containing the egg cells to ripen and several of these stimulated follicles come to the surface of the ovary.

3. One of these ripened follicles reaches the surface first, and the surrounding follicle wall, now quite thin, ruptures and releases the egg or ovum. *Ovulation* is said to have taken place.

This event is initiated by a surge in the amount of luteinising hormone (LH) in the circulation. The reason for this surge is as follows: The ripening follicles produce the hormone *oestrogen* and it has a 'negative' effect on the pituitary, gradually cancelling the production of FSH. As the levels of oestrogen in the blood continue to rise it then has a 'positive' effect on the pituitary and a sudden marked rise in LH occurs about mid-cycle. *It is this rise or 'surge' which induces ovulation.*

4. After ovulation has taken place the empty follicle collapses in on itself to form a tiny yellowish-red structure on the surface of the ovary known as the *corpus luteum*. This structure produces the second main female hormone called *progesterone*. Together with oestrogen, this hormone acts on

the hypothalamus and pituitary in a negative way, so that the levels of both FSH and LH fall.

What has been happening to the endometrium during these events?

5. The *endometrium* during the first half of the cycle is stimulated by increasing amounts of oestrogen circulating in the blood. It repairs itself following the previous menstruation, becomes thick and more vascular. This is termed the *proliferative phase*.

6. The endometrium during the second half of the cycle is now influenced by the progesterone hormone. It gets much thicker, is full of glands filled with secretion, and contains many blood vessels giving it a rich blood supply. This is termed the *secretory phase*. The purpose of this change is to prepare a suitable nourishing 'bed' in which a fertilised egg can settle and begin to grow.

7. If no fertilisation has occurred then the levels of oestrogen and progesterone in the bloodstream fall, to reach levels which can no longer sustain the lush secretory endometrium, and so it sloughs off and sheds itself from the uterine cavity as the menstrual flow.

This cycle of changes is complicated to understand. Table 1 seeks to show the sequence of events with the time scale: the timing of the various events is very variable but ovulation always tends to occur 14 days *before* the next menstrual period.

The female hormones

Now let us consider in greater detail the female hormones and what they do. They are of basic importance when their production diminishes after the menopause, and the events just described cease.

There are two main hormones to consider: *oestrogen* and *progesterone*.

Table 1.   Summary of events leading to menstruation

	No. of days
1. After menstruation a follicle ripens: oestrogen is produced: the endometrium proliferates	10
2. Ovulation	
3. The corpus luteum appears: progesterone is produced: small amounts of oestrogen persist: the endometrium becomes secretory	14
4. Degeneration of the corpus luteum: fall in levels of oestrogen and progesterone: menstruation	4
TOTAL	28

OESTROGEN

This is the female hormone 'par excellence'. Its main biological activity is to develop the immature female infant into the mature fully developed female adult. We have already seen that its production is from the ovary. A small amount is also produced by a chemical change of a substance known as *androstenedione* which is produced by the adrenal gland – a structure which lies on top of the kidney.

The actions of oestrogen are chiefly on the following areas:

The genital tract

(a) In all areas, from the vulva, the vagina and up to the uterus, *oestrogen stimulates growth and maintains vascularity*.

(b) *The secretions of the cervix are increased* by oestrogen and this is notably so at mid-cycle so that there is then a favourable environment for spermatozoa.

(c) As already mentioned the *endometrium is repaired* following menstruation *and proliferates* under the influence of oestrogen.

(d) It is likely that the muscular activity of the tubes is increased by oestrogen – again a phenomenon designed to increase the likelihood of fertilisation.

The hypothalamus

It has already been described how rising concentrations of oestrogen coming from the growing ovarian follicle pass back to the hypothalamus and decrease the production of follicle-stimulating hormone – an integral part of the complex events of the menstrual cycle.

The breasts

The full development of the breasts at puberty is effected by oestrogen. The pigmentation of the areola, the growth of the stroma (ground substance) of the breasts, and their system of ducts are all due to oestrogen.

The cardiovascular system

Oestrogen relaxes the muscle walls of blood vessels causing dilatation of vessels and improved circulation. This may in part explain the lower incidence of coronary thrombosis in women.

The skeleton

Oestrogen plays a part in retaining calcium in bones and at puberty produces a growth spurt which then stops earlier than in the male due to the closure of the epiphyses (bone growth areas) of the long bones. Hence girls tend to be shorter than boys.

Secondary sex characteristics

These are some of the other characteristics which reach full development in girls at puberty apart from the changes described above in the vagina, uterus and breasts. For instance, the overall typical female configuration – narrow shoulders, broad hips, thighs that converge, and arms that tend to diverge. Again, the high-pitched voice, the typical distribution of hair and so on.

These are all partly mediated by oestrogen and partly simply by the absence of the male hormone testosterone.

Psychological characteristics

No one could claim that the typical psychology of the female (if there is such a thing) is simply due to the hormone oestrogen. Inheritance, family upbringing, tribal custom – all sorts of influences make the woman what she is. But oestrogens are important: typical femininity – difficult to define but easy to recognise – is influenced by the presence of oestrogens in the circulation. Libido is increased.

Mood changes in women may be markedly influenced by oestrogen and most women know that it is common in the first half of the menstrual cycle to feel energetic, cheerful and optimistic – the phase when oestrogen output is at its highest. When oestrogen output falls away and progesterone increases, the mood may change and, particularly just before menstruation, a woman may become lethargic and quite depressed.

There are other more complex structural and biochemical changes in which oestrogen is involved but for our present purpose the outline above will suffice.

One further aspect of the hormone oestrogen must be mentioned as it will be relevant later in discussing the use of oestrogens in the management of the menopause. There are three types of oestrogen secreted and they are called:

Oestradiol – the strongest oestrogen
Oestrone – this is in equilibrium with oestradiol in the circulation
Oestriol – this is really a breakdown product of oestrone and is the weakest of the three.

Seventy per cent of the oestrogens circulating in the bloodstream are 'bound' to a specific protein and they are finally broken down by the liver to be released from the body in the bile (from which some may be re-absorbed into the blood) and in the urine.

Progesterone

In many ways this second female hormone can be regarded as an anti-oestrogen substance. Its chief purpose is really to prepare for, and help to sustain, pregnancy. As already shown it is produced by the corpus luteum after ovulation and it is also produced by the placenta during pregnancy.

It is finally broken down by the liver and secreted in the urine as its breakdown product, pregnanediol.

The actions of progesterone are chiefly on the following areas:

The genital tract

(a) The endometrium becomes secretory (see p. 25) with many glands.
(b) The cervical secretions are lessened by progesterone.
(c) It diminishes the muscular activity of the uterine wall.

Hypothalamus and pituitary

It inhibits the production of LH (see p. 24), and progesterone injections or the all-progesterone pill (more correctly the word should be *progestogen* – a progesterone-like substance) will prevent ovulation.

Cardiovascular system

It does not have the same effect on blood vessels as oestrogen. It does cause some water and salt retention in the body.

The breasts

Progesterone stimulates the growth of the alveoli gland system.

Psychological characteristics

It has already been mentioned that in the second half of the menstrual cycle when the influence of progesterone is at its highest the mood of a woman may change and she may become quiet, lethargic, moody and even overtly depressed.

These then are the two female hormones and an outline of their chief functions. We have also looked briefly at the female anatomy, the way it functions and how it is influenced by these hormones. This is the situation between *puberty*, when anatomy and physiology together reach maturity, and the *menopause*, when the female reproductive mechanisms cease and some, at least, of the anatomy is altered as a result.

3 · The menopause: what it is and why it happens

What it is

Strictly speaking, the word *menopause* means the stopping of menstrual periods. The time leading up to this event and the variable time afterwards should be referred to as the *climacteric*. By common usage 'the menopause' is used to refer to the whole phase of a woman's life before, during and after cessation of menstruation. There seems to be no good reason for not complying with common usage in this book – so 'the menopause' it is!

Another commonly used phrase is of course 'the change of life' or more briefly 'the change'.

This 'change' may go on for a variable length of time – anything from one to five years – and covers a complex of symptoms and bodily changes most of which, but not all, are due to the failing production of oestrogen.

AGE OF THE MENOPAUSE

In the United Kingdom the average age of the menopause is 50 but the variation is between 45 and 55 years. It was thought that the age of the menopause is increasing but recent evidence suggests that it remains fairly static. There is such an entity as premature menopause where for one reason or another (often unknown) the ovaries fail and oestrogen production diminishes at a much earlier age (even in the 20s). If ovaries have to be removed surgically because of a disease process then, naturally, the menopause will result, since as we now know, from our study of the physiology involved, ovarian function is necessary for the continuation of menstruation and the production of oestrogens.

It is, perhaps, worth inserting here a small but very important comment. If a woman of the menopausal age has had no periods for a year or more and then has a bleed this is called *'post-menopausal bleeding'* and must be investigated by a specialist. One of the commoner causes is an early cancer of the endometrium of the uterus and if it is found it can be treated very successfully. *Such an episode of post-menopausal bleeding should never be ignored by doctor or patient alike, whatever the patient's age.*

HISTORY OF THE MENOPAUSE

There is an abundance of historical myth and taboo about menstruation, but very little, if anything, in literature about the menopause. The likeliest reason for this is that life expectancy for a woman has greatly increased. At the turn of the century, for instance, it was 48 years: now it is about 72 years – well beyond the age of the menopause. In other words, people's interest and attention were previously fixed on menstruation and reproduction and there was not much need for applying myth and taboo to the menopause and after.

Another possibility – and in some ways it obtains in present-day Western society – is that cessation of menstruation, and with it the ability to reproduce, was a completely negative event so far as the whole community was concerned. No one bothered with these older women in the way younger women caught and held the attention of those around them.

In many primitive societies, however, the status of the post-menopausal woman is raised. Margaret Mead (1950) (see p. 110), the great anthropologist, describes how in Bali, for instance, post-menopausal women took part in ceremonies with young virgins where menstruating women of the reproductive ages were debarred. Again, the women of the Rahjput classes in India look forward to the menopause because then they can emerge from purdah, move about freely and acquire a higher status in society.

In the United Kingdom – indeed throughout the Western world – medical workers have only comparatively recently turned their attention to the menopause. A whole new literature has appeared, conferences are held throughout the world, clinics are set up in individual hospitals – all within the last 10 years or less, and all designed to study this milestone in a woman's life.

The final comment I want to make about the menopause, and what it is, is mainly medical but verges on the philosophical. Should one regard the menopause as a natural event in life, a part of ageing that cannot be avoided, or should we not rather regard it as a deficiency state like diabetes, where insulin is lacking and can be administered to maintain the body's equilibrium? Recent thinking favours this latter approach.

Since it may influence some of what I write in the next section of this book I should perhaps say that I believe that, as so often applies in medicine, the answer is not clearly the one or the other but somewhere between. *Some women reach this phase in their lives, pass through it and into the next phase with little or no trouble. Some women display many signs and symptoms of an oestrogen deficiency state and respond well to having this state explained and treated. But not everyone behaves or responds in the same way so a 'blanket' plan of treatment for everyone is neither sensible nor desirable.*

Why it happens

First, a reminder. The *menopause* is literally, as we have said, the final cessation of menstruation. It may occur abruptly after only minimal change in the pattern of the periods, or gradually, with the periods becoming irregular, usually with longer and longer intervals between. During this time the ovaries are failing, their function is declining. The years over which this takes place and during which the actual menopause is only one event is sometimes called the perimenopause or, more correctly perhaps, the *climacteric*. This word is derived from the Greek – *klimakter*: a critical phase.

As has previously been pointed out, the word 'menopause' by common usage has come to mean the entire phase of this part of a woman's life. In the descriptions that follow – as indeed in the title of this book itself – the word 'menopause' will be used, although frequently the more correct term 'climacteric' should be employed.

At birth, the ovary contains its full complement of oocytes – or egg cells. When menstruation begins and ovulation occurs, as a relatively regular monthly episode, the egg cells are, naturally, gradually used up.

So from birth, when there are on an average 400 000 oocytes, these diminish in number until at age 40 it has been estimated that there are only about 5000 left. Over the next few years the numbers decline still further until none, or only a few, remain. During these last few years the remaining oocytes become increasingly unresponsive to the hormones of the pituitary. The menstrual cycles which may occur are more often than not 'anovulatory', that is, there is no egg production in the middle of the cycle.

To put these events in a more graphic form:

1. Numbers of oocytes greatly diminished
   Oocytes fail to respond to FSH (follicle stimulating hormone)

   ↓

2. Diminishing production of oestrogen

   ↓

3. Failure of negative feedback mechanism to pituitary (see p. 24)
   Increase in FSH and LH (luteinising hormone) levels

   ↓

4. In spite of this, continuing failure of oocytes to respond

This whole process may take from one to five years or even longer. It is complete when the function of the ovary finally ceases. The age at which this occurs is variable but in industrialised societies is approximately at 50 years.

It is important to note at this point that the production of oestrogen does not completely stop. Other sources of oestrogen remain and the main one is by the conversion of the hormone adrostenedione, which has been previously mentioned, into oestrone. Androstenedione issues from the adrenal gland and the amount of oestrone obtained from it varies from person to person but *may be sufficient to minimise or prevent altogether some of the more troublesome of menopausal symptoms.*

What are its effects?

A more detailed consideration of the effects of the menopause will be given in Chapter 4 so only a summary will be given here.

Most books divide the symptoms of the menopause into three broad groups:

1. *Vasomotor*: essentially this means the effects from blood-vessel changes – typically the 'hot flush'.
2. *Metabolic*: essentially this means the effect on tissues and organs such as bones (backache), skin (thinning of vaginal skin in particular) and genital organs (reduction in size).
3. *Psychological*: this includes a whole host of problems under such headings as nervousness, irritability, headaches, loss of sexual drive, insomnia and so on.

A further heading under 'the menopause – what are its effects' should be, I believe, *'none'* and I further suggest that this heading should come top of any list. It is important that women should keep the menopause in perspective, and remember that it has been estimated that only one-third of menopausal women will experience symptoms of any degree of importance to them. One of the good effects of bringing the menopause out into the open, of discussing it freely in magazines and books and on television is that women will inevitably have a greater understanding of this important event in their lives. One of the bad effects is that discussion and writing will inevitably concentrate on symptoms and signs and hardly any emphasis will be given to the fact that none of these may be experienced at all. The same risk will face us in this book too, but so strongly does the author feel about this point that *no apology will be offered in the next chapter for reiteration of the fact that the topic discussed may never be experienced by the individual woman.*

An understanding of the physiological processes, yes; a grasp of methods of treating troublesome symptoms, yes: an attitude of tense, worried expectation – *most definitely, no.* (It is an interesting reflection that before the menopause became 'popular' I used to advise anxious women who might seek a consultation solely for the purpose of knowing 'what to expect at the menopause' not even to learn to spell the word, far less memorise possible problems. Nowadays, such a tritely facetious comment is unacceptable but the basis for it remains.)

Bearing this important message in mind we will now consider in detail what may be experienced by women as a result of the gradual failure of their ovarian mechanism. Abrupt removal of the ovaries at surgery will also cause the menopause to occur and this event will be discussed too.

4 · Menopausal symptoms and signs

First it may be helpful to explain the terms symptoms and signs – words which doctors frequently use and which imply two very different things. A *symptom* is a problem or a 'complaint' which the sufferer is aware of – pain is a symptom, for example. A *sign* is something which is noted by the doctor examining the patient but which the patient may be unaware of – a raised blood pressure, for instance.

On the whole, women approaching the menopause are looking for, or are becoming aware of, *symptoms*. During the course of examining such a patient the doctor will observe any relevant *signs*. In the discussion which follows both symptoms and signs will be outlined without necessarily distinguishing them but it is important to remember the distinction.

Finally, these symptoms and signs are all based on our knowledge, however basic, of the normal anatomy and physiology of the female body. (Hence the *raison d'être* for the first two chapters of this book.)

Let us consider the symptoms and signs of the menopause under the three headings mentioned in Chapter 3. But remember the fourth heading which really tops the list – NONE.

Vasomotor

This word refers to the effects of nerves acting on the walls of blood vessels, causing them either to dilate or constrict. In the case of the menopause the effect is one of dilatation.

HOT FLUSHES

These are the best known of the symptoms of the menopause. A feeling of heat occurs quite suddenly and may involve the chest, neck and face. It is accompanied by reddening of the skin which is obvious to an observer, thereby adding to the discomfiture of the sufferer. They vary greatly in frequency and intensity sometimes occurring only a few times during the day, sometimes several times in an hour. They give the greatest problem when they occur frequently during the night, wakening the sufferer who has to throw off the bedclothes for relief thereby disturbing her sleep. Following the hot flush, a feeling of chill and actual shivering may occur. Perspiration frequently accompanies the hot flush.

The cause of hot flushes is not known for certain but is probably due to a number of factors, low oestrogen levels being only one. They may begin some time before menstruation ceases and continue for several years afterwards but most usually are self-limiting, perhaps because of the continuing production of some oestrogen from sources other than the ovaries, as has been mentioned. (A rare condition, a tumour of the adrenal gland, called a phaeochromocytoma which secretes a substance called adrenalin, produces hot flushes in the same way and when a woman presents herself to a doctor with this particular symptom, this condition will be borne in mind, particularly if the age of the patient is rather against a diagnosis of the menopause.)

PALPITATIONS

These are not infrequently complained of by menopausal women and may occur along with the hot flush. The unpleasant awareness of the heart beating rapidly or even irregularly may be accompanied by a feeling of faintness. Their origin is again obscure.

HEADACHE

This is one of the symptoms of the menopause which will be mentioned again in the psychosomatic group, showing how often menopausal symptoms from each group overlap.

There is no doubt, however, that women in this age group do quite frequently suffer from 'tension' or migraine-like headaches. They are often quoted in medical literature as being part of the picture of 'vasomotor instability' which appears at this time. The term 'vasomotor instability' is somewhat vague but implies exactly what it says, namely that the nerve control and therefore the behaviour of the blood vessels is unstable.

These vasomotor effects are not only the symptoms, par excellence, of the menopause but because of their effect on the sufferer create a number of other problems which will be mentioned later. *They are also the symptoms most amenable to treatment.*

Metabolic

This word is used to describe the way in which cells, structures and organs of the body maintain their function. Perhaps it is too wide a term to use for the subjects discussed below but it will suffice.

The changes which occur at the time of the menopause primarily affect the genital tract and its contents and function. These will be discussed first. Other more distant structures also alter and symptoms may result – these will be mentioned also.

THE VULVA

The skin of the vulva may become thin, and shrinkage of the opening to the vagina may occur. The pubic hair becomes more sparse and turns grey. Rarely, atrophy of the vulval skin gives rise to recognised skin problems called collectively *vulval dysplasias* – with soreness, perhaps irritation, and cracking, particularly in the folds.

These striking changes, however, are much more a feature of elderly women, well past the menopause, and once more it must be pointed out that the paramenopausal women will almost certainly not notice any of these changes whatsoever.

THE VAGINA

Thinning of the vaginal skin may also occur but again this is usually minimal in the early paramenopausal years. With advancing age the vaginal skin takes on a typically inflamed appearance, reddened, thin, with tiny spots of haemorrhage under the skin – a picture which is described as *'senile vaginitis'*.

The younger, sexually active menopausal woman may experience dryness at the time of intercourse, with vaginal soreness but this is amenable to treatment. A lubricating jelly, local oestrogen cream, continuing sexual activity with a sympathetic and understanding partner, are the usual ingredients for successful treatment. Painful intercourse is the greatest reducer of sexual drive, and it may well produce a host of psychosomatic symptoms – headache (especially at bedtime!), anxiety, depression, to name a few. This is another good example of the interlinking of many of these menopausal symptoms.

THE OVARIES

We have already examined the events in the decline of ovarian function. Perhaps the most striking result is cessation of menstruation. It has been mentioned that this may occur quite abruptly, there having been little or no disturbance of the periods beforehand. More usually the periods tend to dwindle – getting shorter, with longer intervals between. Heavy, prolonged, irregular bleeding in this 45 to 50 age group must certainly never be written off by the woman as 'the change'. She should seek advice from her doctor and almost always it will be necessary to sample the lining of the uterus (the endometrium) to make sure that no disease, such as early malignant change, is present. Very rarely is such a change found but it must be looked for in such circumstances. The traditional D and C (*dilating* the cervix to enter the cavity of the uterus and scraping or *curetting* out some of the endometrium – a procedure carried out under a short general anaesthetic) may be advised, or quite frequently, nowadays, the procedure can be done using special suction equipment on an outpatient basis without anaesthesia as it causes very little discomfort.

It is worth noting that malignant change in the endometrium tends to herald itself early by an episode of such bleeding and once diagnosed *is eminently treatable and curable*.

The ovaries themselves get smaller after the menopause and in elderly women are very small indeed.

THE UTERUS

Apart from the changes affecting the endometrium which have just been described, the uterus itself gets smaller and in old age may be quite tiny.

The ligaments and tissues surrounding and supporting the uterus may become weakened and result in a prolapse of one form or another. Prolapse is a word which literally means slipping forwards or downwards. Where the uterus is concerned there are varying degrees of this 'slipping' or dropping downwards – the greatest being a complete prolapse or *procidentia* where the uterus appears right outside the vagina. Other types of prolapse may occur with or without much involvement of the uterus. A *cystocele* is a bulge of the front wall of the vagina carrying the bladder with it: a *rectocele* is a bulge of the back wall of the vagina carrying the rectum or lower bowel with it. Prolapse tends to occur in the post-menopausal years in women who have had children, particularly if they have had several, with rather long labours and heavy babies. The weakening effect on the supports of the uterus at the time of the menopause does mean, however, that occasionally prolapse of the uterus occurs in women who have never had babies.

The *symptoms* of prolapse are outlined in Table 2. The *signs* are, quite literally, a bulge seen by the examining doctor when the patient coughs, or, in the case of a marked degree of prolapse of the uterus, a lump protruding from the vagina seen by the patient when she examines herself with a mirror.

Table 2.   Symptoms of prolapse

---

1. A sensation of 'dropping' from the vagina
2. Feeling or seeing a lump appearing at the vaginal opening on self-examination
3. Difficulty in initiating micturition
4. Feeling of incomplete emptying of the bladder
5. Difficulty in defaecation
6. Feeling of incomplete emptying of the bowel
7. Involuntary passage of urine on coughing or straining
8. Feeling of 'obstruction' at the time of intercourse
9. Backache (often associated with excessive weight)

Nowadays treatment is almost always by surgery, the operation being carried out 'from below' involving no abdominal scar.

THE BLADDER

Although not strictly part of the genital tract, the bladder is anatomically closely involved with the uterus and vagina. Not only that but it also has a common origin with the genital tract during the development of the embryo in the very earliest stages of pregnancy. It is not surprising, therefore, that it too may be involved in menopausal changes. Like the vagina the lining mucous membrane may become thin and the bladder 'shrink' in a sense. This may lead to symptoms of frequency of passing urine, urgency (the need to 'get there' quickly) and even urge incontinence (dribbling of urine before the lavatory can be reached). Actual urinary infections may occur, with pain on passing urine and, if a prolapse of the bladder is present, symptoms of 'stress incontinence' may appear. This means that when the woman coughs or sneezes or strains in any way a small amount of urine is passed involuntarily.

None of these problems may arise in the individual woman but when they do a great deal can be done to relieve them. This will be discussed in the following chapter.

EXTRA-PELVIC STRUCTURES

A number of structures outside the pelvis may–*or may not!*–show changes with the menopause, and symptoms may–*or may not!*–result.

The breast

With cessation of the normal cyclical hormone stimulus to the breast, it is not surprising that in the post-menopausal years the breasts become less firm, diminish in size and the nipples, too, become smaller and flatter. This is a gradual process and it is not until old age that the breasts tend to become thin and drooping with the skin rather wrinkled.

These changes do not tend to cause symptoms although some women find them a psychological blow. In this respect a good supporting bra and, for the married woman, the attention of an equally supporting and understanding partner are of great therapeutic value to the 'sagging' morale.

Bones and joints

After the age of 50 women suffer from fractures much more than men, these fractures involving especially the wrists, the hips and the bones of the back or vertebrae. It is also a well-known fact that elderly women seem to shrink, giving rise to the popular literary or theatrical image of a 'little old lady'. This image has its basis in medical fact since there is a tendency for the vertebrae to collapse in elderly women. The cause of this, and of the increase in fractures after the menopause, is the loss of bone substance or thinning of bone (osteoporosis is its correct name). It has been estimated that loss of bone mass after the age of 50 occurs at the rate of 3 per cent for about six years and then 1 to 2 per cent each year. Of course, not every woman has this precise degree of osteoporosis but, potentially, this loss of bone substance could be the most significant of all the problems of the menopause. In the elderly a fracture of the hip can often be fatal.

It has clearly been shown that small doses of oestrogen can prevent or minimise osteoporosis, the only problem being that oestrogen treatment must be continued indefinitely otherwise the problem will return. Equally, once osteo-porosis has occurred to a significant degree it cannot be reversed by giving oestrogens. So there arise problems in treatment which are still a source of controversy. Should women be given oestrogens indefinitely because of this possible problem of osteoporosis? Such an idea carries problems since, as we will see, oestrogen therapy is not without its risks in the long term. Further scientific investigations are needed to clarify this point but one fact seems to be clear: loss of bone substance is particularly accelerated if the function of the ovaries ceases before the age of 45, e.g. removal of the ovaries at the time of hysterectomy. Therefore there does appear to be a place for giving oestrogens to such women and for continuing the treatment for some time, although the exact duration must still be a matter of personal opinion.

One further and much simpler point must be made. Exercise and a good diet containing plenty of calcium and vitamin D will help in maintaining bone structure. It goes without saying that this is a much more natural and 'healthier' approach to the problem.

When the ovaries cease to function there appears to occur an increased laxity of ligaments and a reduction of muscle strength. It is not too difficult to understand how this could give rise to various aches and pains, especially in weight-bearing joints such as the ankles and knees, in the shoulders and in the back. The small joints of the hand may also be involved. But the problem is that as the years advance, 'wear and tear' on joints is inevitable and arthritis may develop. It is difficult to know whether many of these complaints are due to hormone deficiency or not. It is fair to say that some studies have shown an improvement in symptoms following oestrogen therapy, but here again merely to treat such problems arbitrarily with oestrogens would be wrong without first looking for other causes. Again, healthy living with exercise, proper diet and, particularly, avoidance of overweight must play an important part.

The cardiovascular system

This title refers to the blood vessels and the heart: the condition of which we particularly think is thrombosis, and coronary thrombosis in particular.

It is well known that the incidence of coronary thrombosis in pre-menopausal women is small by comparison with men of similar age, and that the incidence rises after the menopause. It seemed reasonable to conclude therefore that oestrogen had a protective action which was lost after the menopause. Unfortunately this has not proved to be the case and although a clear picture of what part oestrogen does play in this important disease has not yet emerged one or two interesting facts are certain. For one thing the risk of coronary disease actually increases at a steady rate throughout a woman's life while a decrease in the risk to the male occurs between the ages of 55 and 65 so that the risk ratio between men and women becomes altered. Again it does seem from the facts available that if a woman reaches a premature menopause, whether naturally or following surgery, her risk of developing cardiovascular disease is increased, so that again there is a case not only for conserving healthy ovaries at the time of hysterectomy in younger women (see p. 85) but for giving such women oestrogen replacement therapy for a time at least.

Against all this we have to remember the association of oestrogens with an increased risk of thrombosis. No woman over the age of 35 years is nowadays encouraged to continue with the contraceptive pill for this very reason. The type of oestrogen used – whether natural or synthetic – age, build, family history and other factors are all involved; and the answer to this problem – for or against oestrogens in cardiovascular conditions – remains to be clarified.

The skin

We have already seen how the skin of the vulva and vagina is affected by diminishing amounts of oestrogen. But what about the skin in general? As a woman gets older, and particularly after the menopause – take 50 as an average age – changes in the skin certainly take place. There is no doubt, however, that these are due not solely to lack of oestrogen, but perhaps more to the effects of ageing itself – 'wear and tear' if you like. It is fair to say that there are no specific changes in the skin exclusively due to oestrogen lack, apart from those described in the genital region. Almost certainly skin changes elsewhere are due to a combination of ageing and oestrogen lack working together on this most vulnerable structure.

Most of the changes are well known: the natural resilience and elasticity of the skin diminishes and wrinkles appear; drooping of the skin of the chin and general laxity of the neck region occur. It is interesting that these changes appear mainly in white women and in the areas exposed to light. In old age, women (and men) may take on a 'leathery' look and this is particularly noticeable where exposure to a lot of 'all weather' conditions occurs. The main changes may be summarised as follows:

- the skin becomes dry and flaky and as a result may cause irritation
- patches of thickened pigmented skin may appear especially on the backs of the hands
- nail growth slows down
- hair becomes thinner on the scalp and body. Fortunately extensive hair loss occurs mostly in men. Gradual greying of the hair is a common feature of ageing and will vary from individual to individual. Hair growth in other areas may actually increase, e.g. on the upper lip and chin.

None of these changes is serious so far as a woman's health is concerned but they may cause a considerable degree of upset to the morale of the ageing woman. After all, most women take pride in their appearance and rightly judge their complexion as a major part of their attraction. Lack of oestrogen alone however, it must be re-stated, is not the cause of these changes and so merely giving oestrogens will not reverse them. Women hardly need to be told that other simple approaches can be employed: healthy diet, avoidance of overweight, judicious use of make-up with perhaps the advice of a good, honest, professional beautician from time to time if so desired. For the married woman the continuing loving support and admiration of her partner provide perhaps the most important single factor in maintaining a woman's attractive appearance!

Psychological

Now we must consider the very large group of symptoms which were put under the title of 'psychological' in the previous chapter but because of their complexity should perhaps have the more cumbersome but truer title of *'psycho-social-cultural'*. In other words, the problems which we will now examine are not purely 'in the mind' but are often related more to the social circumstances in which a woman finds herself and to her cultural background.

Probably it is simpler to have a list of the most common of these symptoms first of all, not in any order of frequency or importance.

Headaches
Poor memory
Insomnia
Depression
Feeling of inadequacy
Irritability: 'moodiness'
Frigidity: loss of sexual drive

Not infrequently, women come to consult their doctor or gynaecologist with one or more of these symptoms and they themselves may already have decided that this is due to the menopause and that hormone tablets will help. This can even happen before menstruation has ceased but, nothing daunted, the woman may then say that she is 'entering the change' and again surely hormones will cure. The plain fact of the matter is that while many, if not all, of these problems may indeed be related to menopausal changes, many, if not all, can be produced by external situations totally unrelated to hormone changes. It may be difficult for the individual woman to understand or accept this fact but with insight there is a much greater chance of improving the situation with or without the help of hormones. Fundamental to the understanding of the sufferer is, needless to say, the understanding of her husband or partner, her family and her physician, who will do nothing to help by simply scribbling out a prescription for oestrogens.

Let us look at the symptoms as listed. There are others, but these are a representative sample, and there is no doubt that every menopausal woman reading this book will identify one or more which she can apply to herself.

HEADACHES

This is a very common symptom in any age group. It has a multitude of causes ranging from medical problems such as high blood pressure, true migraine, due for example to allergy to certain foods, and brain tumours (rare) to psychosomatic problems (i.e. triggered off by the mind whether consciously or subconsciously) such as response to stress, anxiety or a need to avoid some unpleasant situation.

Now many women who are at the menopause claim to have headaches as a prominent feature of their symptoms. Very often if such a patient is questioned closely she has always had a tendency to headaches even although that tendency is now more pronounced.

Let me be more precise. There is no evidence that headaches as such are a true feature of the menopause and there is certainly no evidence that giving oestrogens will cure them. Headaches are much more likely to be part of an anxiety state which so frequently appears in this age group, and the understanding doctor having first satisfied himself – and the patient – that no disease process exists must try to help the sufferer to a greater understanding of what is happening. Proper use of simple analgesics is of value, but caution in the quantities consumed of even such commonplace drugs as aspirin and paracetamol must be observed and the good physician will be careful to give appropriate advice.

POOR MEMORY

This is perhaps not such a common complaint among menopausal women but can be very distressing when it occurs. Again one must be dogmatic and say that it is not a result of oestrogen deficiency. Much more is it one of a number of vague symptoms which may arise at the menopausal time of life – lassitude, loss of a feeling of well-being, insomnia and so on. There are many reasons for these and they will be discussed later. In the very elderly, where arteriosclerosis or 'hardening of the arteries' of the brain may develop, poor memory or actual loss of memory not infrequently develops. This is something quite different. In the younger menopausal woman no such event is likely to be happening and equally no tablet of oestrogen – or any other tablet for that matter – is likely to correct this single symptom. It is the author's firm belief that the problem can be tackled by the individual herself in the same way as she can tackle her overall well-being. The mind can be exercised in the same way as the body and it should not be allowed to lie fallow. Read, think, talk; use tricks to remember things, such as mnemonics for shopping lists; use notebooks or diaries to jot things down to be remembered – and so on. In other words keep intellectually active, and perhaps it is reasonable to advise menopausal women *not* to apply to themselves that well-known line of poetry: 'what is this life, if full of care: we have no time to stand and stare'. I know of no scientific evidence for these comments but they work!

INSOMNIA

Again here is a problem which is *not* due to lack of oestrogen but it certainly is a common complaint among menopausal women. There are, I think, two main factors to be considered. First, it *is* true to say that the older one gets the less sleep one needs. Babies spend most of their 24-hour day asleep; children sleep deeply for 10 or more hours after a day of hectic physical activity; adolescents often sleep just as long, even though their night may not begin until the early hours of the morning. But older people may be rested after only six to eight hours of sleep especially if their daytime activity has been limited. So first of all we have to learn to accept that as we grow older less sleep is needed and a frantic rush to the doctor to get a supply of sleeping tablets is not only unnecessary but inadvisable. Of course difficulty in falling asleep can be aggravating and so can waking after only an hour or two and then finding difficulty in getting back to sleep again. Remember simple things: do *not* drink tea or coffee late at night, because they have a stimulating effect; and if the need to pass urine is the problem which wakens you, do not drink anything after, say, six or seven o'clock and make sure that the bladder is completely empty before going to bed.

Secondly, it may well be that hot flushes and sweats are the cause of disturbed nights. They may be a major reason for wakefulness and discomfort to the sufferer and, where she is married, to her partner also – and then friction develops, so that finally separate rooms are decided on which, needless to say, means the end to any happy sexual relationship (surely in itself the best sedative for a good night's rest). Now here at last one can say that oestrogens *will* be of value and any woman suffering from frequent and disturbing night sweats should seek help from her doctor so as to break the vicious cycle as early as possible.

DEPRESSION

This is an over-used word and it is very common indeed for people of all age groups to say that they feel 'depressed' from time to time when what they really mean is that they feel low spirited, 'down', vaguely unhappy. True depression in the psychiatric sense is quite a different entity, compounded of a variety of signs and symptoms often only recognisable by a trained psychiatrist. Unnecessary anxieties, lack of emotional responses, undue fatigue, physical symptoms such as headaches and many other features may be part of a true depression, and if these are a persistent feature of the menopausal woman then she should be seen and assessed by a doctor – but not necessarily by a psychiatrist.

Now this type of depressive picture has been ascribed to the menopause and failure of the ovaries but all scientific studies which have been carried out fail to confirm this. There seems little doubt that the menopause coincides with an age group which is in any case at higher risk of depressive illness. Indeed one extensive study carried out in Aberdeen showed that no depressive symptom emerged completely afresh in the menopause and that there was always some past history of a depressive type.

Other factors occur at this time in a woman's life and although they may be obvious in the recounting, nevertheless the 'depressed' menopausal woman may not appreciate their significance and may even find them difficult to accept as an explanation for her own symptoms. In the married woman's case her children have grown up and no longer need her close maternal care. If they are adolescents they may be causing anxiety by their behaviour and not infrequently this may result in friction between father and mother when 'sides' are taken. Older children leave home and go to work or college. The break is complete when the children marry and settle elsewhere.

Then again at this age the husband or partner has usually reached the height of his work or professional achievement. This may mean harder work, longer hours, greater distraction, and less time for home and for his now lonelier wife. In a strong, soundly based marriage, these changes may not create significant stress but where the marriage has had a weaker basis before, they may lead to anxieties, depression, sleeplessness and the possibility of marital breakdown.

In the case of the single woman she may be finding the extra pressures of greater seniority and responsibility at work no longer easy to cope with. And she is now at an age where the prospect of marriage, far less a family, has finally receded, possibly leaving her regretful or even bitter.

At this age the parents of the menopausal woman have reached old age and anxieties may arise there. She may have to look after one or both in her own home now, or visit frequently while constantly worrying as to what should be done for the best. For a married woman a busy distracted husband may be of no real help or may even resent the presence of an elderly relative in his home. For the single woman there may be the double burden of work *and* caring for the elderly relative. Another source of stress and anxiety.

And many other 'life situations', as the Americans would term them, can be instanced, all of them occurring really as natural phenomena in the life history of the woman involved and *not* specifically as a menopausal condition or syndrome.

Oestrogen therapy has no part to play in such problems. Insight, understanding, the ability, and indeed facility, to talk to a sympathetic husband or partner or friend are of the greatest value. If the symptoms of 'depression' seem overwhelming then the help of a doctor must be sought. The judicious use of tranquillisers or antidepressants has a part to play but notice the word 'judicious'. Wholesale swallowing of tranquillisers will do nothing without insight, and insight may have to be worked at.

Is there a place for a psychiatrist? The answer is yes sometimes, but a good general practitioner will be able to make that decision after his own initial assessment and treatment, and he will take great care not even to hint that there is any true psychiatric illness to begin with lest he triggers off further anxieties about mental disease.

While I have said that oestrogen therapy has no part to play in such problems, this is not entirely true. What is true to say is that the consensus of medical opinion stresses the need to deal first of all with depressive/anxiety states in their own right and only if there is failure of treatment should oestrogens be used. If along with these psychosomatic complaints there are hot flushes and atrophic vaginitis for instance, then oestrogens should be given for *these* problems although this will not obviate the need to tackle the others in their own right.

Two items of the list closely associated with depression were a *feeling of inadequacy* and *irritability* or *'moodiness'*. These are obviously part of the psychological picture which I have just attempted to paint and I will not discuss them separately. Having outlined the background to many of these psychological difficulties it should now be apparent why one should rather put them under the title of *psycho-social-cultural*. The whole background to a woman's life influences to what degree she may be affected by any of these difficulties.

Where a happy, stable marriage exists, complete in itself without the 'prop-up' of the children; where a woman has been educated or trained for a job which she can look forward to resuming once the children are 'off her hands'; where the unmarried woman is well and happily established in a fulfilling career; where the woman has many friends with whom she shares interests; where she is prepared to adapt herself and re-shape her life with enthusiasm; where she has never lost interest in herself or pride in her appearance – all these and many other aspects of her social and cultural background will virtually ensure that she passes her menopausal milestone with comparative, if not complete, ease. *And if manifestations of true oestrogen lack intervene then help is at hand in the form of hormone replacement therapy.*

FRIGIDITY: LOSS OF SEXUAL DRIVE

This brings us to the last, and arguably the most important, item on our list: the question of sexuality in the menopausal years.

The first thing that must be said is that there is no evidence whatsoever of any decline in a woman's sexual capacity until very late in her life. And that capacity means not only the ability to have intercourse but to reach orgasm.

There is a belief that some women at the time of the menopause experience a resurgence of sexual desire often to an excessive extent, but there is no sound evidence of any 'flare up' of sexual interests in the menopausal years.

Both men and women have a natural decline in their sexual activity as the years progress and this happens almost certainly for a variety of reasons. The male is more absorbed in work and greater demands are made on his energies. He may, of course, be having extra-marital affairs. The woman's degree of sexual activity is almost always directly related to that of her husband or partner and there is abundant evidence to show that 'sex maintained is sex retained'.

Perhaps it is better and gets us closer to the truth to look at sexual interest rather than actual sexual activity. It is true to say that many women submit to their partner's advances without any enthusiasm or even interest so that to look at the 'desire for sex' or libido is a truer way of assessing the situation. Now it is a fact that decline in sexual interest does occur in the post-menopausal age groups, rising noticeably after the age of 60, in contrast to men who show some decline in sexual interest but not nearly to the same extent.

The important point to decide is the reason for this decline. There are several factors:

1. A reduction in oestrogen level may lead to vaginitis with resulting dryness and pain with intercourse (dyspareunia). The discomfort may occur at the time of intercourse and may continue for many hours afterwards. If no treatment is sought or given, the situation gets worse, libido decreases, the frequency of intercourse lessens, narrowing of the introitus gradually begins and finally intercourse becomes impossible. Here is a situation amenable to treatment, usually with local oestrogen creams only but possibly with the additional help of a lubricating jelly.

2. In a stable, happy 'sex-orientated' marriage little difficulty will be experienced and the natural decline of interest in sex will usually occur much later in life and almost, as it were, by mutual if tacit consent. Other interests and pleasures bind the couple together.

By contrast, in a relationship which has been described by American psychiatrists as 'negative', decline in sexual interest undoubtedly takes place earlier and more rapidly.

3. If early sexual experience has been unhappy then the evidence is that sexual interest declines at an early age.

4. There are, of course, women who, even in this day and age, regard intercourse only as a means of achieving pregnancy and when the ability to have a pregnancy stops after the menopause their interest in sexual activities ceases. This is increasingly rare but by no means unheard of.

5. There is a considerable amount of evidence to show that decreasing sexual activity is influenced by such social factors as level of education, full employment, mental health, social class and so on. This is obvious. The woman who is well orientated to life, busy, interested in events, articulate, enjoying discussions with her husband or partner and maintaining a high level of interest in her appearance and general well-being is very likely to be the woman whose interest in sex declines only very slowly as the years go by.

6. And finally one must repeat that every study done on this subject shows that decreasing sexual activity leads to increasing decline in interest which in itself leads to further decrease of activity. A truly vicious cycle of events which may put intolerable strain on a marriage.

And what part does hormone therapy have to play in improving *this* situation? We have already considered the problem of atrophic vaginitis and its treatment by the use of oestrogen cream. Not only that, but if a woman suffers from hot flushes and night sweats this may lead to disturbed nights, fatigue and irritability – hardly the usual precursors to a happy sex life. Oestrogens will help here, and so indirectly may have what has been described as a 'tonic' effect on the sufferer. She sleeps better, she feels better and more energetic – a perfect precursor to a happy sex life.

Without a history of hot flushes or evidence of vaginitis, however, it is doubtful whether oestrogen will help loss of libido *per se*. Then the doctor (and it is hoped that he will be consulted rather than things being allowed to drift along) must consider and probe into other aspects of the woman's life. Is she truly depressed, in which case there may be need for the use of antidepressant drugs? Is her symptom really just her way of expressing a conscious or subconscious grudge or actual aggression towards her partner? In this situation, help in self-understanding is necessary and here a good marriage guidance counsellor is invaluable.

The male hormone testosterone, present in small quantities in all women, seems to be the hormone which controls sex drive. Its use, usually combined in implant form (see Chapter 5) has been advocated by some gynaecologists and has proved very successful. But one must use it carefully and after full discussion with the patient. We have mentioned that hirsutes (hair) may appear in the older woman, particularly on the upper lip, and testosterone may be blamed for this. Many gynaecologists feel that, on the whole, testosterone should not be used and certainly not used indiscriminately.

A summary of this chapter may not come amiss. There may be many symptoms and signs associated with the menopause but, especially in the well-balanced, educated, contented woman who finds her family, sexual and professional life fulfilling, *there may be no symptoms whatsoever*.

When symptoms occur they can be *vasomotor* – hot flushes, palpitations, headaches – or *metabolic*, with changes in the skin, especially of the vulva and vagina, ovarian changes with resultant menstrual upsets, perhaps uterine prolapse, bladder symptoms, bone and joint changes, hair growth changes. A large group of what we have chosen to call *psycho-social-cultural* symptoms may appear, including depression, anxiety, poor memory, feeling of inadequacy, loss of interest in sex and so on.

The first two groups may be amenable to hormone replacement therapy – outstandingly, hot flushes and atrophic vaginitis. The third group is not specific to oestrogen lack and a large number of family and social events which appear inevitably at this age may be the precipitating factors.

Obviously not only may there be no symptoms but where symptoms do exist there may be overlap in all these groups so that appropriate treatment may have to be combined, namely hormonal, psychological, counselling and generally supportive measures. Insight and understanding on the part of the woman and also her husband or partner will go a long way towards alleviating problems or avoiding them altogether.

5 · Treatment of the menopause

A lot of what will be discussed in this chapter will have been mentioned previously but no excuse is needed for repetition. Women are nowadays particularly and naturally interested in what can be done to help them when troublesome problems arise at this age. And not surprisingly they want to know if there is any risk involved in the treatments which can be offered.

Is treatment always necessary?

The simple answer to this is, no. When hormone replacement therapy was first introduced there was, for a time, a vogue for starting it prior to the menopause and continuing it indefinitely. This approach was popularised in the United States but never really caught on in Britain. In a sense it meant that oestrogens were looked upon as the elixir for eternal youth and beauty and surely even the most optimistic woman must have doubts that such a thing exists. Oestrogens are not without potential problems and indeed in some women should *not* be used, so that their indiscriminate use on a long-term basis is neither sensible nor good medical practice.

What is, or should be, always necessary and can be looked upon as treatment, is proper education on the menopause and what it means. The information available to women is now extensive and usually well-informed although regrettably some of the articles to be found in women's magazines particularly, tend to emphasise the use of oestrogens, implying that they provide an answer to most, if not all, of the problems which a woman may experience at this stage in her life. It is to be hoped that a book such as this will give a more balanced picture.

When is treatment helpful?

This has been discussed already in the preceding chapter but it may help to reiterate the important points. The two main problems which are amenable to hormone therapy are *hot flushes* and *atrophic vaginitis* – the thinning of the vaginal skin, which can cause a number of distressing problems.

These respond to, and ought to be treated by, hormone replacement therapy; the flushes by tablets or an implant, the vaginitis by cream alone or with tablets if it is severe and does not respond quickly enough to local cream. The number of hot flushes which women may experience varies a great deal and it may be that if only the occasional transient episode occurs during the daytime and causes no real upset then hormone treatment will not be necessary. After all the flushes are self-limiting and will stop in time – the only problem being that how long it will take cannot be forecast. If, however, the hot flushes occur frequently and become a social embarrassment as well as a private discomfort, and particularly if they lead to disturbed nights and therefore fatigue, irritability and so on, then certainly hormone treatment should be offered. The word 'offered' is used specifically because it is not unusual to find women – and frequently husbands – who are very much against hormone therapy, having doubts about its safety. The risks of oestrogen therapy will be discussed on page 75, and for some women, because of certain medical conditions, oestrogens must not be given.

There are alternatives to hormone therapy for hot flushes which will be mentioned, but it is fair to say that they are not nearly so successful.

What treatment is available and how does it work?

The mainstay of treatment is *oestrogen*. After all that is precisely the hormone which diminishes in quantity as the ovaries fail. We have already seen that the ovary produces three oestrogens: oestrone, oestriol and oestradiol, the most potent of which is oestradiol. When the ovaries finally cease to function you will remember that a small amount of oestrogen is manufactured by the adrenal glands via the substance androstenedione which these glands produce. This is variable in quantity and may suffice in some women to avoid troublesome menopausal symptoms.

The oestrogens which are available for use therapeutically are broadly (and strictly speaking inaccurately) divided into the *natural* and the *synthetic* oestrogens. The so-called natural oestrogens are derived from animal sources, largely the horse – the pregnant mare to be specific. These secrete large daily quantities of oestrogen and provide a remarkable oestrogen factory. The only problem is that these oestrogens, called equilin and equilenin, must be of great value to the horse but there is some doubt as to their benefit in humans.

Natural oestrogens can also be obtained from the urine of pregnant women. Oestradiol should theoretically be the oestrogen of choice but alone it is broken down or metabolised readily by the liver and gut to produce the less active oestrone and oestriol. By modifying it, however, chemically, a more stable compound can be formed and the most active of the synthetic oestrogens thus produced is *ethinyl oestradiol*. This substance is cheap, easy to use and effective and is still one of the most commonly used drugs.

The naturally occurring oestrogens are just as effective but will, needless to say, cost more. In the management of menopausal problems they have become the drugs of choice both in the United Kingdom and the United States of

America. Several preparations are available, some conjugated with other substances for greater stability.

Table 3 gives a list of the commonly used oestrogens and it is only fair on the pregnant mare to say that when her equilin in the form of sodium equilin sulphate is conjugated with sodium oestrone sulphate it gives a most effective drug which is very commonly prescribed.

Table 3.   Oestrogens in common usage

SYNTHETIC OESTROGENS
  ethinyloestradiol (Lynoral)
  dienoestrol
  chlorotriansene (Tace)

NATURALLY OCCURRING OESTROGENS
  oestradiol
    e.g. oestradiol valerate (Progynova)
  oestriol
    e.g. Ovestin
  oestrone
    e.g. piperazine oestrone sulphate (Harmogen)
  oestriol+oestrone+oestradiol
    e.g. Hormonin
  conjugated oestrogens
    e.g. sodium equilin sulphate+sodium oestrone sulphate
    (Premarin)

The choice as you can see is bewildering and there is in fact little to choose between them although now the consensus of opinion is that there is a place for the addition of a progestogen. This will be discussed on page 65.

Oestrogen cream must also be mentioned. This is for local application to the skin of the vulva or more particularly insertion into the vagina where there are problems of atrophic vaginitis. In severe cases oestrogen tablets may also have to be taken but by and large local applications will suffice. Dienoestrol cream and Premarin cream are available as are stilboestrol pessaries. Creams are usually preferred.

Then we come to implants of oestrogen. These are tiny pellets of oestradiol available in three different strengths. Their value lies in the fact that the relative nuisance of taking tablets is avoided, that symptoms are controlled all the time whereas in the dosage regime of oestrogen tablets (see below) hot flushes may return in the days when no tablets are being taken. Their effect lasts for six to nine months, they are usually put into the fat of the abdominal wall – a painless procedure done under local anaesthetic. But once in place nothing can be done to prevent absorption, which is highly variable, and, not only that, they are expensive, so that their use is mainly reserved for patients undergoing surgery, when it is convenient to place an implant in the abdominal wall before the wound is closed. It is probably advisable to give five to seven days of a progestogen each month to a woman receiving oestrogen implants and who still has her uterus – otherwise heavy prolonged bleeding may occur.

Dose regime for oestrogen replacement therapy

Following a complete examination including a careful history of previous illnesses such as liver disease, or present problems such as varicose veins (see p. 80), examination of the breasts, a pelvic examination including a cervical smear test and measuring the blood pressure, the doctor will then decide on the drug to be used and should give adequate explanation of its use, its benefits and its disadvantages.

It is usual to give oestrogens in the smallest dose required to relieve symptoms and to instruct the woman to take it cyclically. This means that she takes one tablet a day for three weeks and then discontinues for one week. The idea behind this is that it is a more natural or physiological way of providing oestrogens to the body than giving a constant dose – although small doses given continuously can and are used especially in women without a uterus. It also allows the 'build-up' effect of oestrogens on such target organs as the breast and uterus to be reduced.

Bleeding from the uterus may occur during the tablet-free week but this is not so common with small doses of oestrogen alone or in older women well past the menopause. If it does occur it must be reported to the doctor and investigation as for post-menopausal bleeding will be carried out by sampling the endometrium to make sure that it is healthy. The only exception to this is where a combination of oestrogen and a progestogen is used and where withdrawal bleeding occurs as a natural event. Since this is the regime most commonly employed nowadays let us consider the hormone progesterone and its place in the treatment of menopausal problems. Before doing so it is most important to say that any woman on oestrogen therapy must be seen and examined by a doctor regularly. In the opinion of the author this should be every six months or, at the most, every year.

A final comment about the duration of treatment. Opinions vary widely about this from the short sharp course of oestrogens to the 'keep young forever' approach – although the latter is, in fairness, much less common now. Holding the strong view that no drugs of any kind should be taken by anyone unless absolutely necessary the author's approach is to treat patients on the regular cyclical basis described above for a year and then begin to 'wean' them off by extending the week off the tablets to two weeks for a month or two, then three weeks and so on. Usually in the course of a further year only an occasional three-week course of tablets is taken from time to time until they are finally stopped altogether. Obviously not every woman responds in the same way and variations in this regime are not infrequently required.

The next hormone which we have to consider is *progesterone* – the second of the two main female hormones. Progesterone by itself or progesterone-like drugs, correctly termed 'progestogens', have no helpful effect in controlling symptoms such as hot flushes or vaginitis. What has been shown to be important, however, is the combination of oestrogen with a progestogen in hormone replacement therapy. There is still some variation of opinion as to whether or not the addition of a progestogen is advisable, but increasingly the evidence seems to point that way. On theoretical grounds alone it would seem to be sensible. By adding a progestogen to the last week of treatment, nature is being mimicked more closely: there is some evidence that progesterone may block oestrogen receptor organs such as the breast and so limit an overgrowth of tissue; and so far as the endometrium is concerned, the 'build-up' which occurs as a result of treatment is induced to shed at the end of each course in the tablet-free week, thus preventing excessive hyperplasia or excessive growth of the endometrium. There is good evidence that the addition of a progestogen thereby diminishes the risk of cancer of the endometrium which unopposed long-term treatment with oestrogens carries (see p. 75).

Dose regime for combined oestrogen-progestogen therapy

Several products are available as shown in Table 4. In most of these the tablets are taken in the same cyclical fashion – 21 days on, seven days off – and the progestogen is contained in the tablets for the last week of treatment. The tablets are presented in a suitably marked package.

Since some women find it difficult to remember the above regime some combined preparations are available to be taken for the complete 28 days without any break,

Table 4.   Combined oestrogen-progestogen preparations

Cyclo-Progynova
oestradiol valerate 1mg or 2mg
levonorgestrel 250 micrograms

Prempak
conjugated equine oestrogens 625 micrograms or 1.25mg
norgestrel 500 micrograms

Menophase
mestranol
norethisterone
These are given in graded doses (see Table 5) throughout the
entire cycle

Trisequens
oestradiol
oestriol
norethisterone
These are given in graded doses (see Table 5) throughout the
entire cycle

proceeding straight to the next packet. These are quoted in
Table 5.

The benefit of this is not only as an *aide-mémoire* but also
that oestrogen is being continued throughout so that
women who may have tried the other regime and found
that hot flushes return, even to excess, in the week off
treatment have that week covered also.

Now how does one choose which preparation to use
among such a selection? First, let it be repeated that those
women who require treatment are those who are troubled
by hot flushes particularly, which can be so disturbing to

Table 5.   Continuous hormone replacement therapy

Tablets Menophase

mestranol 12.5 micrograms	– 5 tablets (pink)
mestranol 25 micrograms	– 8 tablets (orange)
mestranol 50 micrograms	– 2 tablets (yellow)
mestranol 25 micrograms norethisterone 1mg	– 3 tablets (green)
mestranol 30 micrograms norethisterone 1.5mg	– 6 tablets (blue)
mestranol 20 micrograms norethisterone 750 micrograms	– 4 tablets (lavender)

Tablets Trisequens

oestradiol 2mg, oestriol 1mg	– 12 tablets (blue)
oestradiol 2mg, oestriol 1mg norethisterone acetate 1mg	– 10 tablets (white)
oestradiol 1mg, oestriol 0.5mg	– 6 tablets (red)

sleep or social or professional activities; and those who have problems of atrophic vaginitis, leading to painful intercourse and reduction of sexual activity with possible marital disharmony. The many other problems which we have examined, not directly resulting from the above, must be looked at and thought about carefully before simply prescribing hormone replacement therapy. (Notice we should now refer to it as *hormone* replacement therapy rather than simply oestrogen replacement therapy since progestogens are so frequently used in combination with oestrogens. HRT is the fashionable term.) Many women, however, do find an overall tonic effect when they take HRT and so to the author's mind, at least, if a woman who has taken the trouble to inform herself about the subject requests that she should be prescribed HRT then she should be given it—provided, and this is of the utmost importance, that there is nothing in her past or present medical history, or on examination, to contra-indicate it and provided that full and informed discussion takes place between patient and doctor so that the patient is fully aware of potential risks. It is to be hoped that these are not exaggerated by the reluctant doctor—of whom there is still quite a number.

Now as to which preparation to use there is no definitive answer. Almost always nowadays a combined oestrogen-progestogen preparation will be given although older women in particular may find the regular withdrawal bleeding which ensues unacceptable, even after explanation. In such women, low-dosage, all-oestrogen preparations can be used but any bleeding must be investigated as has been discussed. It is also true to say, incidentally, that in women having regular withdrawal bleeds on the combined preparation it is probably wise to sample the endometrium, say on an annual basis, just to keep a watchful eye on the situation.

The dosage of HRT to give is also by no means universally agreed. Common sense tells us that the smallest dose possible to abolish or minimise symptoms is the one required. Some authorities therefore start with the smallest dose available and only increase if symptoms continue. Others start with higher doses and reduce after a time. The author's practice is to assess the severity of symptoms and start on a high or low dose accordingly, reducing the former when symptoms are controlled.

From all that has been said thus far it must be apparent that the assessment of the menopausal woman and the unravelling of her symptoms is quite complicated and certainly time consuming. A sympathetic listener, a thoughtful counsellor, an atmosphere of unhurried discussion – all these can contribute so much to the care of the worried and often despondent menopausal woman. In the context of many busy general practitioners' surgeries it is not reasonable to expect the time required, although many modern health centres have set aside time for gynaecological clinics in which the menopausal woman can be interviewed. In many hospitals, menopausal clinics have been set up and there is little doubt that their value both to the patients and to the furtherance of the understanding and management of menopausal problems is immense.

Testosterone

One further hormone must be considered and that is *testosterone*. This is essentially the male hormone and indeed may produce masculinisation in the female, particularly in respect of excess facial hair.

Testosterone is formed in the female, however, partly produced by the adrenal gland and, in the post-menopausal woman, from the ovary, which seems to secrete far more testosterone than in the pre-menopausal woman. This may explain why hirsutism can develop in older women, with possibly a degree of defeminisation – but this is by no means a regular feature of the post-menopausal years.

Now it has been shown that testosterone will increase libido or sex drive and in women in whom this is a *primary* problem, i.e. not secondary to a painful vagina which should be treated with oestrogens, a small dose of a testosterone derivative has been recommended. This can be combined with oestrogen in tablet form or given as an implant together with an implant of oestrogen. Such preparations are shown in Table 6.

Because of its masculinising effect it must be used carefully although the relief of symptoms may outweigh any disadvantages. It is probable that only the subcutaneous implant is effective in restoring libido and giving an

---

Table 6.   Oestrogen-testosterone preparations

TABLETS
Mixogen
ethinyl oestradiol 4.4 micrograms
methyltestosterone 3.6 micrograms
   Dose: 1 to 2 tablets daily for three weeks out of four

IMPLANTS
testosterone 50 – 100mg
oestradiol 50 – 100mg
These are implanted together into the fat of the abdominal
wall or thigh

---

improvement in general well-being. The results are said to
be apparent in four to six weeks and, like the oestrogen
implant, should remain for six to nine months.

To give a complete picture of therapy that is available for
the relief of menopausal symptoms we should consider
other drugs and make a brief mention again of obvious but
important aspects of therapy which do not employ drugs.

Other drugs used in the menopause

In the next section we will be considering the risks of HRT
and we will see how in some women oestrogens should not
be used. These women may, however, have symptoms such
as severe hot flushes which have to be tackled somehow.

CLONIDINE (DIXARIT)

This is a drug which appears to lessen the responsiveness of
the blood vessels to either dilatation or constriction and is
used for instance in migraine. It has been shown to be of

some benefit in the hot flushes of the menopause and is useful where headaches are a feature.

PROGESTOGENS

It has already been stated that progestogens *on their own* have little part to play in the treatment of hot flushes, for instance. But there is some evidence that given by injection a progestogen may have some helpful effect and the drug that has been used is medroxyprogesterone acetate (Depo-Provera). This is given by deep intramuscular injection every four to six weeks. Progestogens by mouth have been used with some good results reported, but again one must remember their masculinising effect if given for a long time.

ANTIDEPRESSANTS AND TRANQUILLISERS

Regrettably it is true to say that in all age groups throughout the Western world there is excessive use, leading to actual abuse of these drugs. They have become a household byword – a music hall (or TV) joke. Who is to blame? The drug firms certainly, the doctor certainly – but patients themselves must take a large share of responsibility. How often do patients go to the doctor's surgery specifically to seek a tablet to calm them down or to buck them up, because they are either anxious and 'stressed' or 'depressed' and feeling low. Modern life itself must take the main responsibility for all this with its stresses, anxieties and pressures. But do we not create the life we lead, are we not largely responsible for many of the situations in which we find ourselves and should we not be more able to find resources within ourselves to cope rather better without necessarily having recourse to drugs?

We have seen how the menopause can be a time of particular stress to many women, facing as they are the changes which are happening in their family circumstances as well as in their own bodies. A few women will become depressed, in the proper medical sense of this word, and here the use of antidrepressants or tranquillisers will be necessary. But they should be prescribed after proper medical assessment and the help of a psychiatrist may be required. Medically there are really two schools of thought so far as the 'psychological' problems of the menopause are concerned. One group would say that first treat depression, anxiety and their related symptoms with psychiatric support and appropriate antidepressant drugs, and if this fails try HRT. At the other end of the scale, HRT enthusiasts would say try HRT first and if that fails turn to psychiatric help or to antidepressants or both.

As always, in things medical, the answer probably lies somewhere between. If a woman suffers from a number of menopausal symptoms such as have been discussed in this book and if she is lucky enough to have a sympathetic doctor or gynaecologist, or can attend a menopause clinic, then her symptoms will be considered thoughtfully and appropriate treatment will be given.

LOCAL CREAMS AND PESSARIES

The use of oestrogen creams in problems of atrophic vaginitis has been mentioned. It has to be remembered that absorption of oestrogen into the bloodstream will occur from these and with varying results. There are situations where it may be considered inadvisable that even a small amount of oestrogen should be added to the system, e.g. in breast cancer.

One of the problems affecting the vaginal skin as a result of lack of oestrogen is that it becomes more alkaline and loses the acidity which is a part of its protective mechanism against infection. The use of acidic preparations may help to reverse this process, for example jellies (Aci-Jel) inserted by an applicator or pessaries (lactic acid pessaries). These can also be used as an adjunct to oestrogen therapy.

For dryness at the time of intercourse a lubricant jelly such as KY jelly can be very helpful.

PYRIDOXINE (VITAMIN B$_6$)

This drug has been used with considerable success in the problem of the 'premenstrual syndrome'–the situation where a woman becomes irritable, moody, depressed and so on for 10 days or so prior to menstruation. Interestingly enough some investigators have reported similar problems in menopausal women receiving oestrogen therapy, and if this occurs it may be of some help to take pyridoxine along with the oestrogens particularly if mood changes, depression, loss of concentration and so on are part of the picture prior to prescribing oestrogens. In other words pyridoxine may prove to be a useful adjunct to oestrogen therapy or it may be worth trying on its own where oestrogens are contra-indicated. The results of more extensive investigations are needed to show its true value.

Other therapy

No excuse is given for repetition here! To summarise:

1. Women should learn to understand the menopause more, by reading and by discussion. Be informed, not just depressed by old wives' tales. Treatment *is* available for symptoms but understanding is a most important factor both in the treatment and prevention of symptoms.

2. Women should in many ways make preparation for the change that will inevitably occur in their personal and domestic lives. A job, hobbies, social activities should all be planned. For the married woman greater interest and involvement in husbands' work and activities.

3. Attention to diet. Weight gain is *not* inevitable at this age provided that it is remembered that the older one gets the less food one needs or should consume. Fresh

vegetables, fruit, fish, meat and fewer carbohydrates give a healthy diet high in vitamins and calcium.

4. Exercise. This is good both for avoiding excessive weight gain and for keeping muscles and joints in good 'trim'. Walking and keep-fit classes are both valuable sources of exercise.

5. Women at the menopause should take a special interest in their appearance. Hairdressing, cosmetics (used with care and skill) and clothes are all important aids to appearance and to raising personal morale.

6. Finally, for the married woman, if life seems bereft after children have left home and the stark facts of a shaky 'husband and wife alone' situation face the menopausal woman then she should try very hard to re-establish a sound and even strengthened relationship with her husband. He has his problems too. Talk (not excessively!) – communicate, is probably a better word – re-establish mutual interests and most of all maintain a mutually satisfying and enjoyable sex life even if oestrogens or lubricants or whatever are necessary. Life has to be worked at, not just allowed to happen – and this is never truer than at the time of the menopause. Early widowhood may face the menopausal woman as an extra burden. Here is a subject in its own right but family, friends, work, may all help to tap resources of inner strength at this difficult time.

Let me end this section by re-stating that, to the author at least, it seems to be more sensible to regard the menopause as a milestone in life. Nevertheless one must respect those who think it is a deficiency state requiring administration of the deficient substance, namely oestrogen. The answer lies almost certainly in preparing for this stage in life and if no problems arise – and this is often the case – then it is a bonus. After all no periods mean less 'bother' and, after a time, mean no contraceptive precautions (see p. 81) so that sex life can become less inhibited and more enjoyable. Older age brings greater experience and greater wisdom, if you like – fewer unnecessary anxieties.

If symptoms do arise then treatment is available and this treatment is successful in almost every case.

The risks of hormone therapy

No drug therapy is without its risks, its adverse side-effects, and hormone replacement therapy is no exception. The intelligent woman will not want to start such treatment without knowing something about its disadvantages so that she can balance those against the advantages of the therapy.

When we consider the disadvantages we are really discussing oestrogen therapy since progestogen seems to carry very few problems and indeed, as we have seen, may be helpful in avoiding some of the problems of oestrogen therapy alone. Before looking at the main problems involved one has to stress that as so often in medicine there may be no clear answer to give or picture to paint. This is something which the lay person sometimes finds difficult to accept, or even annoying, but that is the situation and often it has to be left to the doctor to weigh up any evidence that is available and to make a decision about treatment accordingly.

Cancer of the uterus

There does appear to be a definite increased risk of developing cancer of the endometrium (the lining of the uterus) with oestrogen therapy. The chance of any woman developing such a cancer is about one in a thousand – the risk is increased to an estimated four to eight per thousand when oestrogens are taken. But to keep things in perspective it must be remembered that smoking increases the risk of lung cancer by an estimated 17 times.

Many studies have been carried out to try to determine the exact relationship, but not infrequently they have had to be criticised for omitting to take into consideration other possible influencing factors such as age, previous menstrual history, obesity, nationality and so on. What do seem to emerge from the welter of literature are these facts:

- there is an increased risk of endometrial cancer with oestrogen therapy
- that risk is related to both long-term oestrogen therapy and fairly high doses of oestrogen
- progestogens appear to have a 'protective' effect by blocking the action of the oestrogens on the endometrial cells (although not diminishing its overall clinical efficacy)

It seems reasonable to conclude, therefore, that low-dose oestrogen therapy used in interrupted courses, preferably in combination with a progestogen for a limited time and under close supervision, is safe, and its advantages for those who require it certainly outweigh its disadvantages.

The problem of bleeding during treatment has been mentioned. This can sometimes be avoided by altering the dose or the compound used. The regular shedding of the endometrium induced by incorporating progestogen into the last week of each cycle of treatment is thought to be an advantage. Nevertheless this potentially important warning sign must be investigated in its own right. Bleeding during treatment must be investigated and many authorities would favour sampling the endometrium from time to time even in those women who seem to have simply regular progestogen withdrawal bleeding.

CANCER OF THE BREAST

This is an obvious source of anxiety to women who are

reaching the age of increased incidence of breast cancer anyway. It can be stated from all the investigations that have been done so far that there is no evidence of an increased risk of developing breast cancer if the newer low-dose oestrogens are used, possibly with the help of added progestogens. If there is any increased risk it is marginal and related to unopposed oestrogens being used for extended periods of time.

Again it can be said that women requiring HRT to alleviate symptoms can take it with confidence but under close supervision and that supervision should include regular breast examination.

DEEP VEIN THROMBOSIS AND THROMBO-EMBOLISM

The first three words refer to blood clotting in deeper, more major veins such as the deep veins of the calf; the last word refers to the breaking off of a piece of clot which may then travel to a distant site where it can cause blockage of a vessel and resultant damage to the organ involved – for example, the lungs, the heart, the brain.

Most authorities agree that there is an associated risk between the oral contraceptives and blood clotting problems. There is much less agreement on whether a similar risk arises with the small doses of oestrogen used in HRT. The consensus of present opinion is that there is *no* increase in the incidence of thrombo-embolic disorders with low-dose hormone replacement therapy. At one time it was thought that there might be a difference between synthetic and 'natural' oestrogens in this respect – the former causing a greater risk – but there is in fact no real evidence to support this view.

Oestrogens undoubtedly cause changes in the blood, affecting the factors concerned with the clotting mechanism. Although there is no need for a woman to fear the risk of thrombosis by taking HRT, nevertheless if she has a past history of thrombosis her doctor would be justified in not exposing her even to this small extra risk.

HIGH BLOOD PRESSURE

Quite simply, there is no association between oestrogens as given in HRT and any significant rise of blood pressure. There is, therefore, no reason why a woman should have this treatment withheld from her *if it is clearly needed*.

Because we know that oestrogens, as used in the oral contraceptives, are associated with a rise in blood pressure in a significant number of women and because it seems that some women respond to conjugated oestrogens with a rise of blood pressure it is, however, important that all women on HRT should have their blood pressures checked as part of their routine supervision.

GALLSTONES

From all studies that have been carried out it appears that women taking oestrogens after the menopause have a two and a half times higher risk factor of developing gallstones compared to women of the same age group not on oestrogens. Again, to keep the situation in perspective the incidence of gallstones requiring surgical removal in women aged 45 to 49 is quoted as 87 per 100 000 per year – in the HRT group of the same age it is 218 per 100 000.

Summary of risks v. benefits of HRT

These then are the chief risks, and knowing these we must now balance the risks against the benefits. Various complicated statistical analyses have been used to do this but they are not particularly applicable to a book such as this. The majority of women simply want to know what most gynaecologists and doctors believe. Here is an attempt to summarise present thinking.

1. There is no justification for giving hormone replacement therapy indiscriminately to all post-menopausal women. On the other hand the informed woman requesting treatment should probably not be refused it provided that there are no health reasons to contra-indicate it.

2. There may be a place for giving HRT routinely to all women who have undergone a premature menopause whether surgically or naturally. There is a lot of evidence to favour this approach and some of it has been mentioned.

3. If menopausal symptoms are clearly related to oestrogen lack – hot flushes and atrophic vaginitis – then HRT is indicated. To deny it would be quite wrong unless definite medical contra-indications exist.

4. If symptoms are less easily definable, then there is a place for closer analyses of these; discussion with the woman, or with husband and wife in the case of the married woman, so that a clearer picture of both domestic and personal background can be obtained, and referral for psychiatric support if genuine depression seems to be present.

5. In all women given HRT, low-dose, short-term therapy should be the aim with careful supervision throughout. Cyclical treatment, probably best using a progestogen with the oestrogen, is advisable and any abnormal bleeding must be investigated.

6. All patients on HRT must be regularly supervised with cervical smears, breast examination and blood pressure checks.

7. *Absolute* reasons for *not* prescribing HRT are:

 – known or suspected breast or uterine cancer
 – abnormal uterine bleeding which has not first been investigated
 – past or present thrombosis
 – liver or gall bladder disease

Relative reasons for considering carefully, before prescribing HRT:

- a family history of breast or uterine cancer
- severe varicose veins
- high blood pressure
- diabetes
- fibroids
- obesity and heavy smoking

In the final analysis there is no uniform recommendation that can be made which is applicable to all women. Each woman must be assessed in her own right and the decision must be hers guided by her physician. But of one thing there is no doubt, and that is that the use of HRT can and does greatly improve the quality of a woman's life when she reaches the menopause and experiences problems truly related to oestrogen deficiency. This knowledge should provide a source of optimism to a woman approaching the menopause but should not, I trust, prevent her from thinking about, understanding and tackling the other aspects of her life which will change at this time and which can be such important contributory factors to many menopausal problems.

6 · Questions which arise at the menopause

Many questions come to the mind of the menopausal woman and most of these have, I hope, been answered. What happens at the menopause, how will it affect me, what am I to expect, what treatment is available, how effective is it and is it safe?

But there are other medical questions which arise and in the author's experience they mainly relate to three things:

1. Can contraception be safely stopped at the time of the menopause?
2. If a hysterectomy is necessary what does this mean and what effect will it have?
3. Are regular 'check-ups' necessary after the menopause: what form should they take: how often should they be carried out?

Let us take each one of these and attempt to provide an answer.

Contraception

Most women are nowadays aware of the fact that after the age of 35 they should not take the combined contraceptive pill. The amount of oestrogen contained in the pill is higher than in hormone replacement therapy and there is an association with a higher incidence of thrombosis. Because most women after the age of 35 do not wish to have more children it would mean continuing with the pill for many years and this is obviously not sensible. By the time the menopause has been reached, therefore, other forms of contraception are being used – the coil, the cap, the sheath. Some, either wife or husband, will choose to be sterilised.

Fecundity declines quite rapidly in the years prior to the menopause but as it can never be forecast for an individual when the menopause is going to occur no reliance can be placed on this physiological fact and some form of contraception must continue to be used.

Pregnancies have been reported after the apparent menopause, so it seems possible that an egg may be shed even after periods have apparently ceased. It seems sensible from the evidence available that some form of contraception should be used until at least six months have passed since the last period.

The methods available for women in this age group which are safe and effective are:

1. The coil. If one is already in place, leave it for six months after the last period.
2. The vaginal diaphragm or cap, used together with spermicidal creams, gels or foam is a most useful method at this age. It is effective if used regularly and carefully, it is 'non-invasive' – in other words there is nothing in the uterus itself which might cause abnormal bleeding (such as the coil) – and no drug effect is present.
3. The sheath or condom. If a couple are used to this then it, too, is satisfactory but if not, then it is better for both partners that the vaginal diaphragm is used. The sheath reduces sensation and if vaginal soreness is present it may well aggravate it.
4. The progestogen-only pill may be used in older age groups and is effective with minimal or no side-effects. Irregular bleeding may be a problem, however, and this could be a cause for concern in the paramenopausal age groups. The other methods are better.

Hysterectomy

Removal of the womb (hysterectomy) is most likely to occur in older women if it is to be required at all. Many women have a great fear of losing their uterus, not only because they are naturally apprehensive about surgery but also because they have come to believe (often with the help of 'friends') that the operation will lead to all kinds of undesirable changes in their bodies, their minds and their lives.

Here is a straightforward summary of the facts.

THE REASONS FOR HYSTERECTOMY

There are a number of reasons why a gynaecologist may have to recommend hysterectomy:

Cancer of the uterus

This is an obvious reason and no one would quibble with it. Hysterectomy is mainly carried out for cancer of the endometrium but may be advised for pre-cancerous conditions of the cervix or neck of the womb or for early actual cancer of the cervix.

Fibroids

These are benign tumours of the muscle of the uterus. If they are small and are not giving rise to symptoms they can be ignored but if they are large, producing a noticeable swelling in the lower abdomen or associated with pressure symptoms (for example on the bladder) or heavy menstruation, then in the woman past childbearing years it is sensible to carry out hysterectomy rather than a more conservative operation. Such a conservative operation is called a myomectomy and the fibroids are shelled out and the uterus reconstituted. But this is only possible if there are few fibroids, and because there is a tendency for them to recur myomectomy is a somewhat pointless operation in older women.

Heavy menstruation (menorrhagia)

Everyone has a different idea of what constitutes a 'heavy period' but certainly if large clots are passed, if menstruation becomes prolonged and especially if the woman becomes anaemic as a result, then this must be regarded as abnormal. Fibroids may be the cause, or frequently it is due to an upset in the smooth running function of the menstrual process – so-called 'dysfunctional uterine bleeding' – for a reason that is not entirely clear. This situation is quite different from irregular periods, which as we have seen may be a feature of the approach of the menopause.

In older women in the paramenopausal age group the onset of heavy prolonged menstruation requires investigation and almost certainly a D and C will be advised either done in hospital under a short general anaesthetic or by sampling the endometrium using the fine aspiration curette on an outpatient basis (see p. 41).

If no disease is found in the endometrium then treatment may be given using progestogens, usually for 10 days premenstrually, or non-hormonal treatment is often now tried using a drug called danazol which inhibits the secretion of pituitary gonadotrophins (LH and FSH).

An important point must be made here: a D and C is an investigational procedure, *not* a curative one in this type of problem. Occasionally following a D and C the periods seem to settle down for a few cycles but almost always the menorrhagia (heavy periods) will return. Women quite frequently ask for a D and C when they run into problems, under the misapprehension that this procedure is the cure – it is not.

If conservative treatment fails then hysterectomy may have to be advised and most usually women who have been plagued by troublesome periods find such relief afterwards that all their fears of the operation prove groundless.

THE OPERATION

Hysterectomy is classified as a major operation in the sense that minor operations are very brief, cause little or no trouble to the patient and can often be done on an outpatient or day-stay basis or at the most requiring only a few days in hospital. A D and C is a minor operation. But hysterectomy is, if you like, the 'stock in trade' operation performed by gynaecologists, usually completed in under an hour, more often than not accompanied by no complications whatsoever. In this sense it is probably more sensible to regard it as an 'intermediate' procedure.

Hysterectomy simply means removing the womb itself, including the neck of the womb or cervix. Most usually it is carried out by making an incision into the abdomen but if there is a degree of prolapse, i.e. 'dropping' of the uterus, then it may be carried out by the vaginal route which avoids an abdominal scar. This route can only be employed if the size of the uterus is not unduly large and if the reason for the hysterectomy is a non-malignant one.

The most common incision used for hysterectomy nowadays is the 'bikini' incision which is a transverse incision just above the pubic hairline and below all but the briefest of bikinis. So an ugly scar need not be a worry to the woman facing hysterectomy. Obviously if the uterus is very big–enlarged, for instance by many fibroids–then the gynaecologist may have to employ an 'up and down' incision.

The main question which worries women who have to undergo hysterectomy is whether the ovaries will be removed at the same time. It used to be the policy of gynaecologists to take the age of 45 as the dividing line. Hysterectomy before that age meant leaving the ovaries: after that age they were removed. Nowadays a more conservative attitude is adopted. After the menopause, and especially if hysterectomy is being carried out for malignancy, the ovaries are removed. Before the menopause, and provided that the ovaries are found to be healthy at the time of operation, they are conserved and will therefore continue to function, producing hormones normally. A patient who has had her ovaries conserved will not, therefore, experience sudden menopausal symptoms. It is always worthwhile discussing with the gynaecologist beforehand whether or not the ovaries are likely to be removed. And indeed there is really no reason why a woman should not express her own preference in the matter – provided, always, she listens carefully to the advice of her gynaecologist.

THE AFTER-EFFECTS OF THE OPERATION

Hysterectomy is like any other operation and for the first day or two there is discomfort. But with modern anaesthesia and pain relief after surgery this is kept to an absolute minimum. Mostly an intravenous infusion – a 'drip' – is set up in theatre when the patient is asleep and will be kept running for 24 to 48 hours until the patient is fully recovered and drinking fluids normally.

Modern management after surgery means that the hysterectomy patient will be out of bed and encouraged to move about the day after surgery. The length of stay in hospital is usually about 10 days. On returning home it is sensible to take life easily for two weeks. A 'long lie-in' in the morning, a rest in the afternoon and early to bed, is probably the best regime to adopt. Housework, cooking, shopping, driving the car are not recommended for these two weeks but full mobility in the house and perhaps short walks in the fresh air will help to speed the patient's return to normal strength. After the two weeks of convalescence are completed more activity can be undertaken but heavy housework, tiring shopping and the like are best avoided. Every woman responds differently and the best guide as to how much activity is undertaken is the way the patient feels. To be easily fatigued is common and is probably nature's way of asking the body to stop and rest.

An examination after six weeks is usually arranged by the gynaecologist, who checks that the abdominal wound has healed and that the top of the vagina, which has been reconstituted after removal of the cervix, has also healed. Thereafter return to normal activity is encouraged. For women who have a job, two months, sometimes three, off work, are necessary.

Intercourse can be resumed after the six-week examination – but the gynaecologist (who may not always remember to comment on this) should be asked specifically. An important point must be stressed here. Although the cervix has been removed, the vagina is reconstituted and, when healing is complete, is of normal capacity. Sexual intercourse therefore is unaffected. Obviously the woman who has undergone hysterectomy frequently feels nervous of being hurt or of damage being done by intercourse but she can be reassured. Gentleness and understanding on the part of her partner will quickly restore normal relationships.

Many women fear the onset of sudden menopausal symptoms after hysterectomy. If the ovaries have not been removed they can be reassured on this point. If the ovaries have had to be removed in a woman who has not yet reached the menopause then hormone treatment therapy may be given if problems arise and provided that there is nothing specifically against such therapy (see p. 75). Very often an implant of oestrogen will be inserted in such a patient before the abdominal wound is closed.

Another misconception about the after effect of hysterectomy is obesity. It is commonly thought that the woman will automatically grow fat once her uterus is removed. This is not so. Overweight comes from eating more food – as well as the wrong food – than that person requires and we have already seen that the older a woman gets the less food she will need. Sitting around after any operation is conducive to 'nibbling' and this may well trigger off excessive weight gain. Simple and sensible dieting is all that is necessary as a prevention.

Hysterectomy is not, therefore, the drastic operation that many women dread and it will not produce dramatic ageing changes in their appearance or general well-being. Many women undoubtedly have a deep-rooted feeling of losing their femininity if hysterectomy is carried out. This is not so but it may take a lot of understanding and discussion on the part of both patient and gynaecologist before she will readily accept the operation. If of course the operation is to be done for a serious condition then persuasion has to be quite forceful in such cases, as time is of the essence. In most women, fortunately, acceptance of the operation is much easier and if they have had a long spell of heavy periods with associated anaemia, such is the relief felt in the long term that a not infrequently heard comment is 'why did I not have it done years ago?'

Routine screening tests

It is understandable that as women grow older the more they become worried about the possibility of cancer. The same happens to men. Women are fortunate in that the two commonest sites for cancer to develop – the breast and the genital tract – are amenable to easy access and examination. Routine examination and screening tests are therefore sensible as part of a 'prevention is better than cure' approach to life. There is no need to become obsessional or neurotic about it. Regular attention to one's teeth is an accepted part of most lives – why not, therefore, regular attention to these other easily reached parts of one's anatomy? Every encouragement is given to women to attend for such examinations – either at their own doctor's surgery or at special well-women clinics. The only reservation is that 'cost-effective' studies in the UK have indicated that five-yearly cervical smears are adequate whereas most gynaecologists would feel that every one to three years is more realistic.

Cervical smears (which will be described more fully later) should be started by the age of 25 years if intercourse has been taking place, and continued to the age of 65. Obviously variations in this will depend upon any abnormalities which may develop.

BREAST SELF-EXAMINATION

Most doctors and clinics encourage women to examine their own breasts, and instruction leaflets are available. An examination once a month is suggested. The author has certain reservations about this as it does seem to give rise to a measure of unnecessary anxiety but provided that the woman has the back-up of a good screening clinic or her own doctor or gynaecologist then self-examination of the breasts is worthwhile.

Technique

Using the finger tips of the opposite hand feel each breast in turn while sitting up and slightly leaning forwards. Start at the upper outer section of the breast and systematically feel each part.

Obviously any lump should be reported to your doctor who, after further examination, may want to refer you for a specialist opinion. He in turn may simply want to repeat the examination at a later date especially if you are still menstruating. Insignificant lumps vary in size with menstruation and the specialist will want to feel the lump at different phases of the menstrual cycle. Or he may want to refer you for mammography, which is an x-ray of the breast of some value in picking out suspicious from innocent areas.

Finally he may want to biopsy the lump – that is, remove it under a short general anaesthetic for laboratory examination to determine its nature.

OTHER SIGNS TO BE AWARE OF

Although no other part of the anatomy is so amenable to self-examination as the breast, there are certainly a number of signs that women should be aware of and which should be reported to their doctors.

Apart from a breast lump which has already been discussed, *unusual bleeding* is one such sign. The type of bleeding at a period, the duration of time between periods and the duration of the period itself all tend to vary towards the menopause but any marked variation from normal should be reported and an examination carried out by the doctor or gynaecologist. A useful 'rule of thumb' – but remembering that all such rules are made to be broken – which can help to guide one as to whether a menstrual variation is of significance or not is that generally the menopause occurs in one of two ways: either *abruptly*, by cessation of the periods with no material change in pattern beforehand; or *gradually*, by the periods becoming scantier with lengthening intervals between. And it is reasonable to regard any other change in pattern as being sufficiently significant at least to warrant a consultation with your doctor or specialist. There are many kinds of variation but of particular significance are heavier and longer periods, bleeding between periods and contact bleeding, e.g. following intercourse.

Another sign to look for is an *unusual discharge*. Most women have some discharge but if the amount and appearance change and especially if it becomes offensive or bloodstained then it should be investigated. Women are prone to vaginal infection by yeast organisms (monilial vaginitis) which give a thick curdy-white discharge associated with irritation. This can be identified by the laboratory from a swab taken from high in the vagina. It can readily be treated by one of a number of anti-fungal preparations either inserted into the vagina as pessaries or cream, or as tablets taken by mouth. The other main infection is by the *Trichomonas vaginalis* organism which produces a yellowish offensive discharge causing soreness rather than irritation. This is treated by a drug called Flagyl (metronidazole) taken orally by both partners.

If the discharge is bloodstained then this may be of particular significance and a thorough examination and cervical smear test are essential.

After the menopause it is not uncommon for an older woman to develop a slight bloodstained discharge possibly accompanied by vaginal soreness, especially at the time of intercourse. This is usually due to thinning of the skin of the vagina which easily 'cracks' causing the soreness and bloodstaining. This atrophic vaginitis as it is called is treated by the insertion of local oestrogen creams or pessaries but must, of course, first of all be examined and a smear taken, to make sure that no other problem co-exists.

Frank (obvious) bleeding occurring one year or later after the menopause is known as *post-menopausal bleeding* and requires full investigation since it may well indicate an early cancer of the lining of the cavity of the uterus. This is a sign which must be reported to the doctor at once. Investigation will include not only a pelvic examination and smear test but arrangement for a 'scrape' of the womb—the D and C (dilatation and curettage)—which will allow a proper inspection of the endometrium to be made by the laboratory. A cancer of the endometrium is commonest in women between the ages of 50 and 60 and responds well to treatment by removal of the uterus and ovaries, with or without a course of radiotherapy before or after surgery.

Another sign which would lead any woman to her doctor

would be an *increasing swelling of the lower abdomen*. This may of course simply be due to excess weight gain but if the swelling is very much localised to the lower abdomen without weight gain being apparent elsewhere then it should be looked into. Fibroids may enlarge to this extent but the swelling may be an ovarian cyst. This is important because although many of these cysts are benign we have to assume that they are malignant and remove them as soon as possible. Unfortunately cancer of the ovary does not provide us with early clues as to its existence so that any swelling of the ovary in the post-menopausal age group means immediate removal. Cancer of the ovary is treated by removal of all the pelvic organs, and surgery is followed either by radiotherapy, if the disease was localised, or by chemotherapy, i.e. drug therapy with potent anti-cancer drugs over a period of time.

Finally, in elderly women, *any persisting sore or ulcer on the vulva* must be reported. Cancer of the vulva is a disease of the elderly and must be watched for especially in those women who are already suffering from one of the vulval dysplasias, i.e. changes in the skin of the vulva due to age and hormone imbalance. A part of the skin may become cancerous and such women need regular examination and if necessary a biopsy taken of a suspicious area.

CERVICAL SMEARS

These still provide the cornerstone of screening tests for women. Sometimes referred to as Papanicolaou smears after the Greek gynaecologist who first described their use, they are of the utmost importance and value. They are usually carried out every three to five years between the ages of 25 and 65 or before or after these ages if it seems appropriate. The test is simple from the patient's point of view and is taken during the course of a gynaecological examination.

A speculum is passed gently into the vagina and the cervix exposed. A wooden spatula is then wiped over the surface of the cervix and the 'discharge' and cell debris thus obtained smeared evenly on a glass slide. The slide is immediately put in a 'fixing' fluid so that it can be sent to the laboratory for careful microscopic examination.

Not only may frank cancer of the cervix be detected by inspection of the cells on the slide but pre-cancerous changes also, and this gives an ideal opportunity for preventive action to be taken.

If an abnormal smear is found then the patient will be referred for specialist opinion. One of two actions may be taken.

1. If there is a suspicious appearance to the cervix then the patient will be admitted to hospital for an examination under an anaesthetic, and a biopsy taken from the area. If there is a cancer then treatment may be either surgery or radiotherapy. Treatment of cancer of the cervix is complicated and is beyond the scope of this book.

2. If the cervix looks normal then a further confirmatory smear may be taken and depending on this result either the patient will be admitted to hospital for a cone biopsy of the cervix carried out under a short anaesthetic, or colposcopy will be done as an outpatient and tiny pieces of suspicious areas taken for laboratory examination.

Cone biopsy entails a piece of the central part of the cervix – shaped rather like a miniature ice cream cone – being removed and the cervix sutured back to a fairly normal shape afterwards. The part removed is sent for microscopic examination by the laboratory.

Colposcopy is a more modern approach to the problem of the abnormal smear. In this procedure the cervix is exposed as for taking a smear and its surface examined by a type of microscope which magnifies to such an extent that the cell structure can be examined. Any abnormal areas can be biopsied with no or only minimal discomfort to the patient. Thereafter, depending on the laboratory report, the abnormal areas can be destroyed, again during inspection by the colposcope and using either cryocautery (freezing to destroy the unhealthy tissue) or a laser beam. Either method is perfectly comfortable for the patient and avoids admission to hospital and the necessity for an anaesthetic.

These then are some of the important modern methods available to women to screen for cancer of the female organs or pre-cancerous conditions. We have also discussed some of the abnormal symptoms and signs which no woman should ignore and which require specialist attention. Women are fortunate in that the organs most prone to disease are so accessible to examination and testing with minimal discomfort.

7 · Personal viewpoint

A lot of what has been written in this book is repetitive, and quite deliberately so. Repetition helps understanding and clarifies ideas. This short chapter is intended to gather together almost all of what has been said in one section of the book or another and present it as the author's personal approach to the menopause. Not everyone, especially other gynaecologists, will agree, and again each individual woman must come to terms with her own feelings about the menopause helped, it is to be hoped, by a sympathetic doctor, by loving family and friends and maybe to some extent by books such as this.

A word of warning. Try not to listen to the tales of well-meaning but interfering friends or relatives. Their information is often gloomy and invariably false.

Growing older is inevitable but with age come a whole host of advantages. For the married woman her family have grown up and make less demands upon her. Indeed, increasingly she can sit back and allow them to 'take over' a bit more. Her husband has usually reached the peak of his career and this brings financial security. For the single woman her career has become established and she too may have reached a position of importance with resulting social and financial benefits. Of course a milestone has been reached and there can be no going back, but the future can be just as full of interest and activity and indeed excitement. Children marry and grandchildren appear. Husbands approach retirement and together new plans can be laid for that era of life.

It is easier for a woman who has had a job previously and can resume it to maintain interest and *joie de vivre* at this time of life. The menopausal woman left at home with nothing to do now that her family have gone and her husband is preoccupied with his career, is the one most likely to suffer, thinking too much about herself, her health, her appearance and the void that seems to stretch before her.

So far as her health is concerned, especially with regard to menopausal symptoms, nothing may happen and to sit around waiting for symptoms will only tend to produce a host of neurotic problems based on no physical changes whatsoever.

We have seen, however, that the menopause is due to the natural ending of ovarian function and the production of oestrogens, so in this sense the menopause is a deficiency state which we have already likened to diabetes where insulin is lacking and where giving insulin corrects the situation. If true 'deficiency state' symptoms arise – and I would list these chiefly as hot flushes (first and foremost), insomnia (usually due to the hot flushes), irritability (because of the insomnia), atrophic vaginal skin changes leading to pain on intercourse and subsequent loss of interest in sex, and one or two others which have already been outlined in a previous chapter, then like any deficiency state this can be corrected by the judicious use of hormone replacement therapy which nowadays provides a tremendous physical boost to the menopausal woman.

But this is not enough. The older woman well past the menopause can, as we all know, be an attractive, vigorous and exciting person. Approach this phase of life positively. Take care over your appearance, skin, hair and most importantly weight, with the help of sensible eating and regular activity. Take up a job again or get involved with voluntary work. Keep mentally active by reading and conversation. After all, you have all your earlier years of experience to borrow from and social ease and enjoyment should come much more easily. If you are married take a greater interest in your partner's work. Keep contact with family so that you and their home are a joy to return to.

Hormone replacement therapy is undoubtedly a godsend for the genuine sufferer; a lively well-informed mind ready to take up the challenge of the post-menopausal years is an even greater godsend. And it can be achieved, of that there is no doubt.

8 · The male 'menopause'

It has been suggested that a book on the menopause would be incomplete without a commentary on any changes which occur in the male at this stage of life. To apply the word 'menopause' to the male is, of course, incorrect, as we have seen from the true meaning of that word. 'Climacteric' is the better word to use. As a gynaecologist whose work is confined to women, it is perhaps presumptuous to write on this topic. Nevertheless a pattern of events happening to the male when he reaches the late 40s, early 50s of his life has become clear not only from patients discussing and revealing their partners' problems, but from general practitioners dealing directly with men of this age and from such commentaries as appear in medical literature. It is not a subject that has received much attention – certainly not in comparison with the female climacteric which has truly 'hit the headlines' in recent years. Much of what follows, therefore, will almost certainly be controversial and may indeed be treated by any man reading this chapter with disbelief if not downright derision.

The first thing that can be said with absolute authority is that there is no comparable physiological change in the male as occurs in the female. We have seen how the level of oestrogens falls dramatically as the function of the ovaries fails in the female. No such event occurs in the output of the male hormone testosterone. There are therefore no typical physical changes in the male at this age related to diminution of hormone output as there are in the female of comparable age. There are, of course, changes due to ageing – even the male cannot avoid these. Skin changes, joint deterioration, greying and indeed loss of hair are all prominent features but may not arise until later years. Such changes – or it might be better to use the word 'upsets' – as may occur appear to be psychological and the identity of the triggering mechanisms is not always clear. It must be stressed, however, that the majority of men will be untroubled physically or psychologically at this age.

The male in his middle years – and let us take the ages of 45 to 55 somewhat arbitrarily – is often in the most active phase of his career. Financial responsibilities both in terms of his family and his business are frequently at their heaviest. Not only that but the challenges of attaining promotion, of achieving greater seniority may be at their keenest. For success a greater workload is often demanded of him. If this is the case then a lot of his drive and energy is used up in the furtherance or maintenance of his career. He may work longer hours, returning home later and more tired. Gradually he realises that he is losing touch with his youth, that he is not getting any younger, and this may add to his concerns over work and finance and his responsibilities.

In the male these sorts of stress equate very much with sexuality. In the context of a loving secure relationship with mutual understanding and adaptation, no problems may arise. A satisfying fulfilling sex life continues and provides the male, particularly, with release from stress and strain. But it is in this age group and often with such a background of stress that sexual dysfunction may arise. Physically, failure of erection or maintenance of erection, premature ejaculation or failure to ejaculate may all occur. Loss of libido, the desire for sex at all, may develop.

It is not surprising that domestic strain intervenes and his partner may show irritability, 'edginess' or downright condemnation. This sort of response can only lead to a vicious cycle of events, and the physical relationship of such a couple deteriorates. Even with a loving understanding partner the male's sexual prowess may continue to diminish under such circumstances of stress.

What happens then very much depends on the personality of the man, his social and his economic status. He may react in a variety of ways. He may try to ignore what has happened and throw himself into his work even more. His partner who herself may be undergoing climacteric changes resulting in loss of sexual interest may be quite relieved, and so a state of relative contentment develops but without the fulfilment of sexual enjoyment. Occasional attempts at intercourse may cause vaginal pain to the woman who may be developing atrophic changes of the vaginal skin and so attempts become fewer.

Then again his partner may become frustrated and angry and this can only result in greater reduction of his sexual drive and performance. If the man's personality is such that he is unable to work through this time of crisis he may become depressed and develop true psychiatric symptoms – anxiety, and what is called reactive depression. He may sleep badly, he may begin to drink too much, he may gamble.

But another reaction altogether may occur. Losing confidence in his youthfulness and particularly his sexual prowess he may seek reassurance away from his own partner and turn to younger women as a means of proving and reassuring himself. Extra-marital affairs are commonest at this age and there seems no doubt that the excitement of a new relationship and the attraction of a much younger woman are often the psychological stimulus that is needed to overcome any sexual difficulties which he may be experiencing. Not only that but if he is in the middle grades of his professional or business life, 'peer pressure' from above may mean that he feels that it is incumbent upon him to seek extra-marital affairs and become 'one of the boys'.

Sadly, as a result of all this, divorce is at a higher rate in this age group and not infrequently disastrous second marriages take place without the expected happiness developing.

Having read this chapter of depressing facts from which emerges a rather sorry picture of the middle-aged male desperately striving to regain his youth, let us keep things in perspective. This picture is the exception, not the rule. Most men grow in stature, as it were, with age and experience. Family bonds remain strong and couples find new and greater happiness together as they approach older age with its change in life pattern. Plans are laid for years of retirement, families are watched growing up, grandchildren are mutually enjoyed, holidays without family encumbrances are relished and so on.

And since this book is for the woman and her 'change of life', what of her in all this? With greater understanding of herself and her bodily changes at this age, with adequate treatment of symptoms if they arise it behoves her to remember her partner also. To remain attractive, caring, interesting and interested must be half the battle surely. There is no evidence whatsoever that declining sexual enjoyment in the female is inevitable after the menopause. Indeed as we have seen, enjoyment of sex may be re-kindled at that time, when the fear of an unwanted pregnancy has been removed. A happy, contented and physically fulfilled life should be a positive aim rather than allowing fear of the opposite to rule the middle-aged couple. Such negative thinking can only lead to disaster one way or another.

A final word. Where difficulties arise in either or both partners they should be recognised and help sought. Not necessarily by immediately turning to doctors, where regrettably tranquillisers and sedatives frequently are handed out as universal panaceas, but by mutual discussion between partners, by sharing anxieties and troubles and by honest examination of what is happening. In this way lies the greatest chance for developing a closer, more confident and fulfilled relationship for the years to come.

Glossary

adrenals The glands on top of the kidneys

alveoli The collection of milk-secreting cells in the breast tissue

analgesic A drug which relieves pain

androstenedione A substance produced by the adrenal glands which is converted into oestrogen by a chemical change

anovulation Without ovulation

areola The pigmented area of skin around the nipple

arteriosclerosis A condition of thickening of the walls of the arteries

atrophic Thinning or shrinking of an organ or tissue

Bartholin's glands The glands lying on either side of the lower part of the labia majora

biopsy A portion of tissue or an organ removed for examination by the laboratory for the purpose of establishing a diagnosis

bladder The organ in the pelvis which collects the urine from the kidneys

cardiovascular system The heart and blood vessels

carunculae myrtiformes The tags of skin left after 'breaking' or stretching of the hymen

cervix The neck of the womb (uterus)

chemotherapy The treatment of disease by drugs

climacteric The phase of life preceding the final menstruation

clitoris The small, highly sensitive, structure at the top of the vulva

coil The intra-uterine contraceptive device

colposcopy A method of examining the surface cells of the cervix

cone biopsy A cone-shaped piece of the cervix removed for laboratory examination

conjugated oestrogens Oestrogens which are chemically joined with other chemicals to increase their stability

contraception The prevention of a pregnancy

corpus luteum The structure which remains after the egg has been shed from its follicle

cortex The outer coat of the ovary

cryocautery Cautery by freezing used to destroy unhealthy tissue

cystocele A prolapse or bulging downwards of the front wall of the vagina, carrying the bladder with it

D and C 'Dilatation and Curettage'. The procedure often called a 'scrape' of the womb where the lining of the womb is scraped out. Carried out chiefly for diagnostic purposes

decidua The thickened lining of the womb during pregnancy

diaphragm The plastic vaginal device used by the female as a form of contraception

Döderlein's bacillus The organism which is a normal inhabitant of the vagina

dyspareunia Painful intercourse

dysplasia Abnormal tissue development

ejaculation The passage of semen from the penis

embryo The earliest stage of the development of the fetus

endometrium The lining of the uterus

equilin: equilenin Oestrogens derived from the urine of pregnant mares

fibroid   A non-malignant tumour of the muscle of the uterus

fimbriae   The finger-like processes at the ends of the Fallopian tubes where they hang over the ovaries

follicle   The tiny structure(s) in the ovary which contains the ova or eggs

frigidity   Lack of desire for, or enjoyment of, sexual intercourse

FSH   Follicle Stimulating Hormone. Produced by the pituitary gland this hormone stimulates the growth of the egg-containing follicle in the ovary

genitalia   The sex organs

gland   A structure which produces fluid or chemicals

gonadotrophins   The hormones of the pituitary gland which stimulate the genital organs

hirsutes   Hairiness

hormone   A chemical substance produced by a gland which influences distant structures by being carried to them in the bloodstream

hormone replacement therapy   Treatment for symptoms of the menopause in which hormones are prescribed to replace those that are lacking after failure of the function of the ovaries

hymen   The incomplete membrane surrounding the opening of the vagina

hyperplasia   Excessive growth

hypothalamus   The portion of the brain which lies above the pituitary gland and controls menstruation

hysterectomy   Surgical removal of the uterus (womb)

implant   A small pellet of hormone (usually oestrogen) inserted into the fat of the thigh or abdomen

insomnia   Inability to sleep

labia   The folds of skin on either side of the entrance to the vagina. The labia majora are the outer folds: the labia minora the inner

LH   Luteinising Hormone. Produced by the pituitary gland this hormone stimulates the development of the corpus luteum and hence the production of progesterone

libido   Sexual desire

ligaments   Bands or sheets of tissue binding two or more bones together

mammography   A soft tissue radiograph (x-ray) of the breasts

masculinisation   Having the characteristics of the male

menarche   The time of the first menstrual period

menopause   The time of the last menstrual period

menorrhagia   Heavy menstruation

menstruation   The monthly period or flow of blood from the vagina

metabolic   Chemical changes within tissues or body structures

mnemonic   A system for helping the memory

monilia   Fungal organism commonly referred to as thrush

mons pubis   The pad of fat covering the pubic bone

myomectomy   An operation to remove fibroids without removing the uterus

oestrogen   The female sex hormone

orgasm   The sexual climax

osteoporosis   Thinning of bone

ovary   The female organ which contains eggs and produces the female hormones

ovulation   The shedding of an egg from its follicle

palpitations   An awareness of the rapid beating of the heart

Papanicolaou smear The scraping taken from the cervix to examine the cells for signs of cancer

paramenopause The years around the time of the menopause

pessary A medicated vaginal suppository *or* a device placed within the vagina to support a prolapse

phaeochromocytoma A tumour of the adrenal gland producing a chemical substance which raises the blood pressure

physiological Referring to normal bodily functions

pituitary The gland situated at the base of the brain which produces hormones influencing menstruation and ovulation

premenstrual tension A number of symptoms experienced by some women just before menstruation

procidentia A major degree of prolapse

progesterone The second of the female hormones produced by the ovary

progestogen A progesterone-like substance

prolapse Literally a 'slipping forward'. Refers to the 'dropping' of the womb or bulging of the walls of the vagina

psychosomatic A physical problem caused by the mind rather than by a disease process

puberty The transition of a child into a young adult

pyridoxine Vitamin B_6

rectocele A protrusion of the lower bowel appearing as a bulging of the back wall of the vagina

rectum The lowest part of the large bowel

releasing factors Substances produced by the hypothalamus which stimulates the release of the pituitary hormones

sheath The condom or protective worn by the male during intercourse to prevent the passage of sperm into the vagina

sign   An abnormality detected by the examining doctor

smear   See Papanicolaou smear

speculum   An instrument designed to be passed into the vagina to display the cervix for examination, and the taking of a smear

spermicidal   A substance which destroys sperms

stroma   The layer of cells in the ovary in which lie the egg-containing follicles

symptom   An abnormality experienced by the patient

syndrome   A group of symptoms and signs

synthetic   Made in the laboratory rather than occurring naturally

testosterone   The male hormone

thrombo-embolism   The breaking off of a piece of blood clot and its travelling to a distant part of the body via the bloodstream

thrombosis   Formation of clot in a blood vessel

tranquilliser   A drug used to calm an anxious or agitated patient

trichomonas vaginalis   A protozoal organism which commonly causes an infection of the vagina

tunica albuginea   The outer covering of the ovary

urethra   The passage leading out from the bladder through which urine is passed

uterus   The womb

vagina   The muscular tube leading from the vulva upwards to the cervix and uterus

vaginitis   Inflammation of the vagina

vasomotor   Referring to the nerves which control the dilatation or constriction of blood vessels

vestibule   The entrance to the vagina

vulva   The outside of the female genitals

Suggested further reading

Bowskill, Derek and Linacre, Anthea (1976). *The 'Male' Menopause*. Pan Books, London.

Cooper, Wendy (1979). *No Change: A biological revolution for women*. Arrow Books, London.

Evans, Barbara (1979). *Life Change: A guide to the menopause, its effects and treatment*. Pan Books, London.

Llewellyn-Jones, Derek (1982). *Everywoman: A gynaecological guide to life*, 3rd edition. Faber and Faber, London.

Mead, Margaret (1950). *Male and Female: A study of the sexes in a changing world*. Gollancz, London. (see page 32).

Saunders, Peter (1981). *Womanwise: Every woman's guide to gynaecology*. Robert Hale, London.

Stoppard, Miriam (1982). *Everywoman's Life Guide*. Macdonald and Company, London.

Utian, W. H. (1978). *The Menopause Manual: A woman's guide to the menopause*. MTP Press Limited, Lancaster.

Index

anatomy of the female genitalia
      13–22
   Bartholin's glands 14–15
   cervix 16, 17
   clitoris 14
   Fallopian tubes 18
   hymen 14
   labia majora 13
   labia minora 14
   ovaries 18–19
   uterus 16–18
   vagina 15–16
   vulva 13
androstenedione 26, 35, 61, 103
antidepressants 71–2

bladder, menopausal changes 43
breasts, anatomy 20–21
   cancer of 76–7
   effects of oestrogen 27
   effects of progesterone 30
   menopausal changes 43
   self-examination 89–90

cardiovascular system 103
   effects of oestrogen 27
   effects of progesterone 30
   HRT risks to 77–8
   menopausal changes 45–6
cervical (Papanicolaou) smear
      89, 92–4, 107, 108
cervix 16, 17, 103
   effects of oestrogen 26–7
   effects of progesterone 29
climacteric 31, 34, 103
clonidine 70–1
colposcopy 93–4, 104
cone biopsy 93, 104
cystocele 41, 104

D and C 41, 84–5, 91, 104
danazol 84
Depo-Provera 71
depression 51–5

endometrium 17, 25, 104
   cancer of 75–6, 91
   effects of oestrogen 27
   effects of progesterone 29
   sampling of 41, 84

follicle-stimulating hormone
      (FSH) 24, 25, 27, 34, 84,
      105
frigidity 55–9, 105

gallstones and HRT 78

headache 39, 49–50
hormone replacement therapy
      see HRT
hormones, definition 24, 104
   of the hypothalamus 24

'hot flushes' 35, 38
  clonidine for 70–1
  HRT for 60–8
  treatment of 60
HRT 57, 59–70, 105
  risks of 75–80
hypothalamus 22–4, 105
  effects of oestrogen 27
  effects of progesterone 29
hysterectomy 83–8, 105
  after-effects 86–8
  reasons for 83–4

insomnia 50–1, 105

KY jelly 72–3

labia majora 13–14, 106
  minora 14
luteinising hormone (LH) 24,
  25, 29, 34, 84, 106

male menopause 98–102
mammography 89, 106
memory, poor 50
menopause, age of 31–2
  and contraception 81–2
  derivation 22
  effects of 35–6
  historical note 32–3
  signs and symptoms 37–58
    metabolic 39–48
    psychological 48–58
    vasomotor 37–9
  treatment 59–80
  what it is 31
  why it happens 33–5
menorrhagia 84, 106
menstruation 22–5, 26, 106

oestrogen(s) 24, 25–9, 61–8, 106
  and cardiovascular disease 46

cream 62
  effects on female 'psy-
    chology' 28
  effects on secondary sex
    changes 28
  and 'hot flushes' 38
  implants 63
  and osteoporosis 44–5
  replacement therapy 63–5
  types 29, 61–2
oestrogen-progestogen therapy
  65–6
oestrogen-testosterone preparations 70
osteoporosis 44–5, 106
ovary, anatomy 18–19, 34–5,
  106
  cancer of 92
  menopausal changes 40–1
  physiology 22–5
ovulation 24, 106

palpitations 38, 106
physiology of the female organs
  22–30
post-menopausal bleeding 32,
  64, 91
procidentia 41, 107
progesterone 24, 25, 29–30, 65,
  107
progestogen 29–30, 65, 66, 71,
  107
prolapse 41–2, 107
pyridoxine 73, 107

rectocele 41, 107

screening tests 88–9
skeletal system, menopausal
  changes 44–5
  oestrogen effects 27
skin, menopausal effects 46–8

testosterone 57, 69, 108
tubes (Fallopian) 18
   effects of oestrogen 27

unusual bleeding 90
   discharge 90–1
uterus, anatomy 16–18
   cancer of 75
      hysterectomy for 83
   effects of oestrogen 26
   effects of progesterone 29

menopausal changes 41

vagina 15–16, 108
   effects of oestrogen 26
   menopausal changes 40
vaginitis, treatment of 40, 56,
      57, 62–3, 72, 108
vulva 13, 109
   effects of oestrogen 26
   menopausal changes 39–40
vulval dysplasias 40, 92, 104